Healing through

T0008090

"Vickie Dodd is one of the true pioneering figures in the field of sound healing. Her work is brilliant—she is a monumental healer who uses sound and an exceptional teacher whose work embraces the true embodiment of sound. Now, finally, for those who know her extraordinary wisdom and abilities, she has produced a book. It's what we've all been waiting for. *Healing through Sound* encompasses all the important aspects of how our own sounds can be used as a transformational and therapeutic modality. Enjoy this amazing journey into the world of sound healing with Vickie Dodd as your guide. You'll be glad you did. Get this book now! It is a most important addition to anyone's library."

~ **Andi and Jonathan Goldman,** sound experts
and authors of *The Humming Effect*

"Vickie Dodd, in her journey as a physical and spiritual healer, has gathered the results of the decades of her creating, searching, and re-searching into this magnificent book of full-body, sound, rhythm, and heartful meditation. As a body percussionist, poet, and vocalist, I have embraced wholeheartedly the whole-force physical, mental, and spiritual exercises she has shared in this book and found them to be transforming. Her call for awakening to the entire energetic field has been heard and felt, and I have responded."

~ **Brenda Bufalino,** jazz and tap dancer,
choreographer, singer, and poet

"The titles of the chapters and their content vibrate at the higher expectations of this advancing new age. Vickie Dodd's well-drenched understanding of sound as a solution for real honest healing supports our readiness to shift more committedly to the creative and intentional use of sound and sounding as a personal and interpersonal sustainable health practice."

~ **LARAAJI,** musician and founder of Ananda Ashram

"I have been in the healing arts field for several decades and I had dabbled in sound such as mantras and Om, but I had never thought of using sound or my voice for my own physical and mental healing. This work that Vickie Dodd is presenting is helpful to anyone in the healing arts. On almost every page there are workable, easy-to-understand tools and methods that can aid anyone. This is a workbook, a textbook, and a roadmap to profound, breakthrough techniques for healing others and self. For the past few months I have been using my voice daily to release stress and align my emotional well-being. My voice is teaching me."

~ **Ralph "Corky" Matson,** body-mind consultant and author of *Prodigious Son: A Memoir of Miracles*

"This is a masterful work deserving of a place in every library committed to the authentic exploration of sound as an essential healing modality. Vickie Dodd is not only a pioneer in this field, but one of the most authentically unique and powerful of its voices. In a time when so many superficially explore this terrain, her integrity and alignment with Divine Source make it a higher calling and a true North Star for any serious student or practitioner seeking genuine wisdom and guidance."

~ **Arji "OceAnanda" Cakouros,** sound healer, musician, and Usui Reiki master

"I have been experimenting with sound healing on and off for years with singing bowls and more. . . . Even so, nothing prepared me for the experiences of healing I received as I began implementing Vickie Dodd's sounding tool as outlined in this book. Her work and guidance has opened up a whole new connection to myself in the present. I hummed, I toned, I followed her teachings as I read. I learned, I grew, and I surrendered as the tones began to tone me, unraveling my stress and traumas and taking me to a deeper acceptance of myself. I believe that this book is a must-read for all who seek to embrace all of themselves, all of life and its infinite possibilities. The tool? Our own voice."

~ **Janet Hudonjorgensen,** energetic healer

Healing through
SOUND

Awakening Your
Audible Body

Vickie Dodd

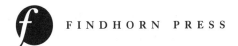
FINDHORN PRESS

Findhorn Press
One Park Street
Rochester, Vermont 05767
www.findhornpress.com

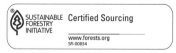

Text stock is SFI certified

Findhorn Press is a division of Inner Traditions International

Disclaimer
The information in this book is given in good faith and intended for information only. Neither author nor publisher can be held liable by any person for any loss or damage whatsoever which may arise from the use of this book or any of the information therein.

A CIP record for this title is available from the Library of Congress

ISBN 979-8-88850-031-6 (print)
ISBN 979-8-88850-032-3 (ebook)

Printed and bound in the United States by Lake Book Manufacturing, LLC. The text stock is SFI certified. The Sustainable Forestry Initiative® program promotes sustainable forest management.

10 9 8 7 6 5 4 3 2 1

Edited by Nicky Leach
Text design and layout by Anna-Kristina Larsson
This book was typeset in Garamond, Fertigo Pro and Avenir Next
Illustrations by Vickie Dodd and Shutterstock (p. 110 ©Tyron da Gama;
p. 111 ©Fascija)

To send correspondence to the author of this book, mail a first-class letter to the author c/o Inner Traditions • Bear & Company, One Park Street, Rochester, VT 05767, USA and we will forward the communication, or contact the author directly at **www.sacredsoundworks.com**.

Scan the QR code and save 25% at InnerTraditions.com. Browse over 2,000 titles on spirituality, the occult, ancient mysteries, new science, holistic health, and natural medicine.

Contents

Chapter 9
Sound as a Spiritual Solution 151

Bali: Sing a Love Song to Your Shadow 151 | Loving Our Many Characters 154 | The Spiritual Significance of Music 159 | The Power of Sound and Vibration Being Made Visible 161

Epilogue
The Mythology of Awakening the Feminine Divine 165

Appendix 1
Additional Sound Vocabulary 168

Appendix 2
Dr. Joseph Liss 170

Appendix 3
Rest Assured: Parasympathetic Resonance Album 171

Foreword
by Rosemary Gladstar

Sssh! Don't bother me. I am reading *Healing through Sound,* and I am fully enthralled!

Reading this book is like reading poetry; it *is* poetry—powerful, deeply moving words that flow together in rhythmic timing. There is a story woven into these pages that tells of family history, of place, of feelings, dreams, and experiences that shape a person. They are sung, and if one listens, one can hear the sounding, sacred sound in the words.

I found these stories powerful as they tell of the sensitivities so many people experience but don't understand, and the un-ease this causes in the psyche. Woven throughout the stories and poetry that comprise *Healing through Sound* are healing exercises and sounding practices one can easily do to help shift patterns, facilitate healing, and ease the disharmony and disruptions that lodge in our beings. This is both a book that inspires and also informs. It gives us simple tools, easily learned, that help us heal our bodies, our souls, and others with sacred sound.

I've had the great good fortune to know the author, Vickie Dodd, for well over 35 years. It was quite apparent from the moment we met that here was an exceptional individual. Vickie was visionary. Long before sound work was recognized in this country, she was using sound to shift and change patterns to heal. She understood sound healing from a deep place within, guided by her own intuition and instincts, and later instructed by some of the most well-known healers of the time. In the ensuing three decades, Vickie has become one of the most recognized healers and teachers of sacred sound healing and has traveled the world over instructing people how to use their voices and their own unique sound to heal from within.

Her work is profound.

I remember a time in the gardens at Sage Mountain, my home in Vermont, when Vickie came to teach sacred sound healing to a group of herbal apprentices. We were walking through the gardens, when Vickie, very quietly and intently, approached a large stone lying in the path. With little ado, she leaned down and placed a hand on either side of the stone. Soon a strange, unfamiliar sound poured forth as she began to tune into the energies of this stone.

It's very hard to describe what happened next, and quite honestly, if there weren't a number of people standing with me who saw and witnessed the very same thing, I'm quite sure I would have thought it was just a figment of my imagination. But we all witnessed it, together, and saw with our own eyes that very stone change shape and form, rearranging itself, as Vickie sang to it.

More recently, when my son and grandson were killed in a tragic accident, and I was bereft and lost in the deepest grief, thinking I would never rise again, Vickie reached out and offered to do a series of sound healings for me. Though we lived miles apart—thousands of miles, in fact—Vickie found the closed pathway to my heart, and through a series of sound healings, done long distance, was able to open my shattered heart, just a little at first, enough so I could see the light of day.

Slowly over a period of weeks, as the sound deepened, my soul began to sing again. It takes time to move from such deep grief, to even want to move from it, and there were a multitude of tools and healing gifts that helped me along the way—flower essences, herbal teas, and long soothing baths; touch and bodywork; thyme and more time, and, most healing of all, the love and support of family and friends. But without a doubt, the sounding that Vickie offered, even from so far away, even without ever seeing her, penetrated to my core and helped shift the patterns of the deepest pain and grief so that I could at least begin, slowly, to dream again.

As Vickie writes in *Healing through Sound*: "All that has ever occurred in our life gets recorded in our bodies. The years of working with clients that I could not physically touch with my hands strengthened and demonstrated to me that Sound alone is Bodywork."

Healing through Sound brings Vickie's story forward, instructs in the practices of sound healing, encourages us to be still and listen. Through it all, if one listens deeply, one hears a sweet hum in the background . . . the sound of listening.

Rosemary Gladstar is the godmother of the herbal renaissance in this country. In 1971, she started the California School of Herbal Studies in Sonoma County. She located and gathered herbalist elders from around the globe to teach young, aspiring herbalists the power, medicine, and respect to be found in nature, as these elders were going to fade away with their knowledge not shared. We are grateful for her insight and courage to awaken the wisdom of the plant world for so many. She is the author of 12 books and the director of Rosemary Gladstar's The Science and Art of Herbalism: An Outstanding Herbal Home Study Course. For more information, visit www.scienceandartofherbalism.com.

Preface

Why We Sound

Sounding Is a Teacher

We sound to wake up.
We continue sounding to stay awake.
Sound is a means to remember.
A tool to dissolve the amnesia . . .
Of what we may have forgotten.
What is our most important vision and mission this life?
Yes . . . it is to wake up!
We sound to quiet the noise in our heads.
The noise that keeps us from being able to listen
to our most important teachings.
The noise that clouds our memory, our thinking.
The noise that creates confusion and miscommunication.
It is not about how good our "chops" are . . .
But how well and willing we are to listen to our Soul's teachings.
Why else are we here if not to listen to what our Soul needs from us,
To complete its mission or cycle?
A call to Awaken.
A call to demystify common sense,
to be restored to what has always been.
Remembering we are made from the minerals of this very Earth.
We sound to clear the noise, even temporarily . . .
To receive our teachings. We sound to listen.
We sound to remember, what has been forgotten.

Sound as an Evolutionary Possibility

When I speak of sound, I do not separate sound, light, color, and movement. Although they can be broken down individually, in my experience they are the same, translating as different octaves, vibrations, and resonance of each other. Sound breaks up crystallization. Sound creates a resonance so that movement starts to manifest, and the reverberation continues. Sound is a definitive tool, a medium for the inner terrain of the physical body, a conduit that is 70–80 percent fluid with an electrical current running through it as the generator.

Sound work is dynamic in nature. It always creates change. When we are exploring our inner bodily terrains, our bodily laboratories, we want to notice where there is pulsation and rhythms and where there isn't. Where there is rhythm, we match its resonance and then follow the pathway it takes us on, and where there isn't resonance, we can use our voices to begin awakening the numbness to discover its unique pattern or rhythm.

The Hum, a method and exercise referred to often in the book, provides the strong foundational work. Practiced daily, the Hum softens and keeps the passageways throughout the body liquid. The Hum employs consonant sounds, allowing it to resonate in the body, creating a reverberation and massaging of the inner landscape. For this method to work, consistency is a major component. It is in the process of doing, tracking, and noticing what occurs that we start learning how sound works within us. Using ourselves as a laboratory allows us to learn this firsthand.

I spent many years daily using sound, Humming and Emptying my noise, my chatter. "Emptying" is an aerobic sounding that creates and activates an inner bodily movement. Examples of Emptying and Humming will be taught throughout this book. I spent weeks, months at times, sounding places of numbness, of amnesia, before I could feel a small movement, a reverberation, an awakening begin to happen. By using my voice, I started waking up the sleep, waking up the deadness, waking up the rhythms of denied expression.

My first years of sounding and doing research in my own body laboratory, I did emptying sounds. I had many layers of congested, embedded, emotional buildup inside my body. I later started naming this as "undigested emotional material." Sounding is a wonderful medium to dissolve stuck unexpressed emotions, especially the held expressions of fear, grief, and anger. I was using my voice to dissolve this formation, which was clouding my ability to listen into my inherent wisdom.

Also, I was doing this to stay awake, as my view of reality was that it was easy to fall into sleep, numbness, as the pain of awareness can be very great at times. Especially in those early days, I was feeling quite alone in this awareness of the need to awaken. These were the early days of the mind–body movement and therapies. In the late 1960s and early 1970s, I knew no one working with sound, and I didn't have any support for sounding.

My soul was my authority and teacher during these years. I started training in massage, acupuncture, shiatsu, and Rolfing. I became an Aston Patterning Movement teacher, studied nutrition, herbalism, and more. I needed assistance for my body and emotions. I also needed to be received as a trusted practitioner to begin listening to bodies and to commence this deep study of listening and sounding.

One of the first teachings that Sound offered
was "that which is unexpressed runs the show."
We sound that which is denied expression.

For the past 50 years, I have maintained a teaching practice and a bodywork practice with sound. I have listened to thousands of stories contained in our bodies. Through this work, I have observed that we all experience some degree of body–mind amnesia.

For example, with clients in the late 1980s, I started noticing an increase in the mucilaginous substance around the cervical spine, a sticky liquid surrounding the nervous system. I do not know what this means, just an observation. I also observed that sounding the cranial area would increase fluidity in the mucilaginous quality.

We want to remember and keep emphasizing that our work with sound is a teaching of evolutionary possibilities. We are wanting and desiring to take the risk that evolution is possible.

In fearful times—which seem to be most any time—we go toward maintenance, the status quo ("Just take the pain away, please."), and our healing sessions can easily become about managing pain. Listening to thousands of bodies taught me that pain is not necessarily the place to look for the source of the problem or the solution. We must always look at the entire being, from head to toe. Physical, emotional, psychological, and spiritual—which "body" is in pain? Which body needs support? What calls us to listen? What memory or feeling wants to be sounded now?

I need to go deeper to the root of the discomfort, a reminder that the motive here is evolution, not maintenance. We may need to notice how much of the allopathic paradigm we have taken on in our traditional studies, possibly without our awareness. In our sound healing paradigm, we ease the discomfort through sound. Our voice creates movement within our liquid terrain, our body. Inner movement in the tissues and cells relieves discomfort and creates a feeling of more ease and connection. We are resourced, naturally!

We sound to create more liquidity in the tissues, to dissolve that which may impede our spiritual and emotional progress.

Seeds of Sound Frequency

My soul has much to do in this life. One of my inner assignments was to travel following ley lines throughout the United States, Latin America, and Northern Europe. I was instructed to plant "Sound Seeds of Encodements." These sound seeds were planted to stimulate encodements, or vortexes, which were inherently ready to wake up. Sounding activated them in their own language.

Sound awakens, and now was the time for another awakening. I walked, drove, and flew for a good 10 years, sounding the earth in the USA, Mexico, and Europe. I sounded large groups in circles of 50–100 people at a time. I did walking meditations, chanting Sound Seeds. I did not "know" what I was doing on an intellectual level. I only knew that it was my "job," and I felt like an obedient worker and journeyer.

This began in 1965, years before sound would be recognized as a frequency medicine or known and remembered as a shamanic form of working within many cultures, as a transformational tool for healing and change.

Sound is my teacher; I do not teach sound.

I was given a teaching through a vision at the top of Monte Alban in Oaxaca, Mexico, in 1966. I was shown in a vision that this land had been a powerful healing site, the site of an ancient hospital. The healing methods used were sound, color, light, movement, and dance. My inner knowing confirmed that sound, color, movement, and vibration were the essential ingredients of all our ancient medicine, and that the roots of the performing arts are the healing arts! Then I was shown the currents, the rootlets, which connected this modality all over the planet.

I was given the confidence that I was "plugged into" an ancient form, and part of my job was to bring it forth. One could never have known how this form of frequency healing was going to take off in the decades that followed. The visionary experience touched my very essence and reverberated through me. My cellular memories were all "enlightened," as an awakening of my record-keeping system was plugged into the Earth matrix memory on Monte Alban. That powerful three-day vision guided and held me confident on my pioneering path during those first 20 years, introducing and planting Seeds of Sound Frequency as a means of therapy.

Root Patterns

Let us go into our own roots, embracing and trusting our own rooting. Accept what is ours, accept our own lineage. If we embrace our roots, we will touch all the rootlets and roots of all others, our entire human *mycelium*. What were the rhythms and root patterns that you were born into?

The Root Patterns

I am from a
boogie-woogie mama,
a two-stepper
with a bluesy voice.
A gambling-gypsy daddy
With black-slicked hair
Who smelled of plumber's oil.
Half-breeds Shawnee—tinkers
And Black Irish . . .
So mixed up and meshed
No one remembers, really
Storytellers—who knows what the truth is or was?

Rowdy people, colorful folks—
Lotsa music . . .
Lotsa beer . . .
Lotsa catfish . . .
Lotsa fear . . .
Lotsa worry . . .
Lotsa fights.
Then the flight for freedom began. Trouble ahead, trouble afar,
Many jails . . .
Really from the beginning.
Held hostage.

Come from roots of hard-earned living,
Poker playing rhapsodies
Wise old women.
Wart removers
Tongue chasers,
Heart answerers
Feet soothers,

Teeth pulled,
Whether they were ready or not—

Lived and grew under the kitchen table.
Listened to the women tell their dreams.
Come from prophesies.
Come from meanings for everything.
Drop a knife—a man's coming,
Right hand itch—you going to get some money.
Dream of death, a baby is coming.
Come from meanings.

Come from poke greens smell so bad,
cook them for hours, maybe days,
smell up the house and neighborhood.
Cooked with side pork that had to be soaked for days and
always cornbread.
Come from food,
Rich food
All local.
Always made every day.

Come from ice boxes and coal heating stoves
and sharing my bed with Grannie . . .
And our room was always the dining room,
the room you'd walk through.
I come from no doors.
I come from a basement my brothers and I made into a fishing hole.
I come from oak trees
And walnut trees
Where I learned to be healed.
I come from folks that laughed at what made you cry
And cry at what made you laugh.

I come from my egg of a cell being in the womb of a woman that
was going to be sold off to her first husband at 11 years.
I come from a woman who prayed when I was in her womb that
I would be light skinned and that I would not have her life
and that I would speak my mind—
I come from grandmas that could see
and they scared me when I
was in my mama's belly
as they could see that life would be what
they didn't know yet.

I came from wisdom of many senses.
I came from a people who hadn't been industrialized
or medicated out of their knowing.
I come from folks who were going to forget
what they knew—very quickly.
And they were going to demonstrate with their own sacrifice
how easily amnesia comes and we start thinking
Walmart is a good choice for a community store.
I come from people that could see the politics of ages.
I come from socialists and Wobblies.
I come from angry folks that didn't get heard.
I come from folks that loved me, and I got to live long enough that
I got to love them.
I come from grace. It took a while for hate to be transformed.
I am grateful that this is possible.

The Lineage of Sound Healing

The Teachings of the Grandmothers

I was born in Eldorado, a small town at the southern tip of Illinois: a place of Wobblies, miners, rivers, drunks, half-breeds, with the flavor and feel of the Ridge of the Ozarks. There was still much Earth wisdom and common sense alive in the inhabitants. We might say, because of its location and economic status, it was a good 25–30 years behind most of America, a place that was mainly untouched by much of the industrial revolution of the 1940s.

My earliest memories of women as healers began around the kitchen table. I played and listened from underneath the table, to the local women who met at my folks' house to have my mom bobby-pin their hair, while they would visit and gossip and smoke their corncob pipes and chew their tobacco. There were few places where that was an acceptable or permissible act.

The women lived their lives according to their dreams. They always seemed to know when another woman was pregnant, and if it was going to be an easy or difficult birth. They said they could tell by their eyes (we now call this iridology). Their dreams would tell them when someone was going to die. I remember my grandma grieving when her husband got killed in a major mine disaster. She told how she'd begged him not to go, as she knew he wouldn't be coming back. But the women's dreams and feelings weren't much listened to; they were referred to as old wives' tales.

Grandma Baggott

My first memory of direct experience with these healing abilities was with a woman called Grandma Baggott. For one year, I had a wart growing inside my mouth, on the underside of my lip. We had been going to our new doctor in town for nearly a year, once a week, for various treatments to burn it off. Nothing was getting to it. On our last visit to Dr. John, he told us we'd have to go to a hospital in a town 80 miles away to have it surgically removed.

Now, going to a doctor was a new idea, and going to a hospital was a shock to the system. We were walking home and met Grandma Baggott at the main corner. Mom told her what was happening with me.

Grandma said, "Let me see that, honey."

I pulled my lip out and showed Grandma this big wart.

She put her hand on my shoulder and looked me in the eye and said, "Honey, you won't have that tomorrow."

The next morning when I awoke, it was gone, and it never recurred. Thank you, Grandma! I was five years old.

No one in my family was surprised. It wasn't "a miracle," because they already knew it was possible. Grandma had removed many people's afflictions. All that mattered to my folks was that the wart was gone, and we were all relieved to not go to the hospital.

I reflect that going to see Dr. John was more about showing others that we were becoming more modern and a part of the world, more affluent. We now call the work that Grandma did Neuro-Linguistic Programming.

During the many decades when frequency medicine was not being acknowledged, my powerful experience at five years of age with Grandma Baggott helped sustain my "knowing." Molecular structures could be changed with intention, touch, love, and belief—letting go and trusting.

A View from the Porch: Observing What Is in Front of Me

In the early 1950s, we had a doctor move into town and more and more town folks started "doctoring." See, "doctoring" showed that you were or had become more affluent. You could afford to go to town and see Dr. John, rather than go see Grandma Rister.

Now, I spent many days on the porch of this boarding house down the street from us, playing jacks and listening to the old women talk amongst themselves. They didn't seem to mind me visiting at the foot of their rockers.

One day I heard someone say, "You know, it seems to me that the more folks 'doctor,' the sicker they get."

Now they weren't trying to be contrary; they were observing their community from the porch view, and in my listening to them, they taught me the power of observing what is in front of me . . . let me be willing to see what is. They were teaching me to observe.

Do I See the Disconnect?

I was teaching an advanced training I called Evolutionary Sound at the Polarity School in Zurich, Switzerland. I had taught these students over a fairly long period of time, so we were comfortable with one another.

I started ranting and raving: "Can you believe we need science to tell us that it is healthy to walk barefoot on the earth? Can you believe we need science to tell us that nature is healing to the emotional and psychological body? Can you believe we have a name for this—'earthing' and 'forest bathing'? I mean can you believe this?"

Oh, I was so very self-righteous and full of myself, and I guess if the truth be known, I was truly blown away that even many colleagues were impressed with these findings! What was I missing? I thought this was the most obvious, evident part of living, that this was a given.

Well, after my speech, I looked around the room and started hearing, "Vickie, we didn't know; we don't know."

That was one of my most potent teachings and possibly most distressing wakeups. I did not know until that moment how disconnected I was from the disconnection all around me! It now had my attention.

It was exciting to me, as I had landed deep into a place of not-knowing. I always desire to go, to be taken to, where I do not know. That is the evolutionary work and intention of sounding. I do not know what I am going to find or what is going to be revealed.

What had my attention here?

Well, these students are very bright lights—they work deeply in various forms of spiritual and therapeutic processes, and many are highly recognized in their fields of study and work. So what is missing? Are we in danger of losing our ability to connect the dots? Are we becoming a people of less connection with our own nature and our dependency on that which is our nature? Do we truly not notice or acknowledge how we feel when walking in the quiet sanctuaries of old-growth forest or in the city parks with the deciduous trees?

I trust that sounding can reconnect intuitional capacities that get easily lost with our focus being so electronically distracted. We can lose our connection to what we are standing upon. Sound reconnects our disconnection.

One of sound's main teachings is its ability to help us remember our nature—that we are nature, and that plants and trees have a nervous system that is similar and often more complex than our own; that the DNA of the planet is similar to our human form; and that we possibly have much to learn from nature itself. Decades after stating that everything I learned about sound frequencies and electromagnetic fields and much more came directly from the earth, I appreciate that what I said may have been interpreted as metaphorical reference, not a literal one.

My interest lies in how to communicate that which is obvious to me and may not be obvious to others. How can we connect the dots, and become aware of our connectedness, especially to nature? Notice always how things in nature are connected to one another? These things are common sense to me. Get to know your nature!

My inner teaching is now looming bigger than ever in front of me.
The excitement that comes from sounding is that it can
take us to places we do not know. That is the goal.
Sounding can help us remember our nature.

Seeing the World as Energy

From the beginning I perceived auras, could see the shapes of energy, perceived sound frequencies from people's bodies and living matter. This was not considered extraordinary; this extrasensory perception was considered common sense.

My coping response to early life—and to my sensitivities—was to hold my breath until I passed out. My mother and the neighbor women told stories of how it scared my mother, how she'd run down the road to Verdia Rister's house, and they'd put me into dishwater, and I'd come to. I did this until I was about two years old.

I now know that I was a "Highly Sensitive" being. There was no such category at that time, but through my private practice of the last five decades, I now know that Highly Sensitive folks are in a great number!

Simply, I perceived life from the experience of not having enough boundaries or cushioning around my own nervous system. I didn't know it wasn't "my business to be in your business." I did not know for many years how not to take on others' mood states. Just because one can perceive another's mood state or auric field does not entitle one to probe or interfere or take on "what is not mine." This required many years and wonderful teachings and therapy to heal and mend. We discuss many of these teachings and ways throughout the book.

I only know in retrospect that I was bombarded with a tremendous amount of energetics that I could not integrate, assimilate, or tolerate. I am grateful that I come from a culture of earth-based people who didn't medicate or institutionalize or religion me out of inherent wisdom. Many of my clients had such experiences, which created yet another or more layers of confusion, guilt, shame, and grief of not being able to remember what they know.

The Rock People

It was August 1987, and a group of about 25 friends were gathered at a wonderful hermitage in northern Wisconsin. Our group had chosen the hermitage to honor the first Harmonic Convergence, created by Jose Arguelles. The event was to herald into consciousness more galactic light upon this dark-trailing earth. Each day, we engaged in fire ceremonies, sweat lodges, breathwork, and sounding. The trusting camaraderie amongst us was wonderful.

Several times a day, I ran barefoot along the dirt path in the forest to my hermitage cottage. While returning to my shelter on the last day, a fairly good size rock in my path asked me to pick it up. Now, I had been there for several days, and there had been no rocks on this or other pathways. It was as if this rock had been dropped out of the sky especially for me, so I honored its request and packed it home to Chicago.

Within a day of being home, the rock started calling me to lie down and hold it on my diaphragm, my abdomen, my heart. I placed the rock on any area it directed me to. This rock literally took me to bed every day for months. I'd lie down, and it would be on me. It was running my life.

I cannot recall how all of this happened, but my partnership with the rock took me through much regression work that revealed deep elements of my life stories. Releasing many layers of emotional holding, I cried and felt layers of unexpressed grief, pain, and regrets opening to receive deep love and acceptance, mercy, and grace.

On and on, day after day, the rock was teaching me the emotional release work I was going to be sharing with others for the next few decades. This was quite profound, but the experience went much deeper. I was instructed to hold and massage the rock as if it were a human form. By 1987, I had already been sounding people with my voice for some time to effect changes in their fascia, tissues, and postural alignment. Now this rock was inviting me to listen to the shape of its "tissue." I was to hold this solid element of nature with the same grace with which I listened to human forms.

I listened deeply with my fingers and my body so that I could sense the held wisdom the rock wanted to reveal. I was invited to use my voice to sound what the rock was revealing. This rock was bringing me into the reality of its aliveness as a living, breathing being!

So, I started experimenting, listening to the layer that was being presented and sounding what I interpreted, and indeed, the rock literally began changing shape! This teaching from nature blew me away. Through listening, sounding, and massaging this being, I witnessed this stone changing shape, one layer of tissue at a time. The rock became my master teacher.

Needless to say, I started finding rocks that wanted to change—and by the way, not all rocks want to change, and it is not my business to know why. One time, I took before-and-after pictures to confirm my own perceptions. Thank goodness enough people had seen my master teacher before it started shape-shifting. I had witnesses to what I was experiencing.

Tapping the Emotional Rhythm

My family said that I didn't speak English until I was nearly seven years old. I didn't know this, as I understood everyone else. My communication was with the plant world, and I truly thought I was communicating.

Blessed be, my mother got me a pair of tap shoes when I was around three years of age. I knew instinctively how to tap dance. I tapped the rhythms of all of the life around me.

One of the first rhythms that entranced me and soothed my system was my mom's wringer washing machine scooting back and forth. *Shalum shaluk, shalum shaluk, shoosha lo, shoosha lo.*

I loved to tap to this bass line and could easily improvise the in-between notes. I tap-danced everywhere, for anyone. And it was welcomed and gently received. I could tap the rhythms I heard; I could tap the emotional life around me and within me. It gave me a vehicle for expression and literally saved my life, I do trust.

My dance teacher, Miss Marlin, had five students. We toured mental hospitals all over southern Illinois, Kentucky, and Missouri. I loved dancing the emotional rhythms I could perceive from the patients, and I trust they might also have welcomed their rhythms being acknowledged. I will always be grateful that my mother had the "knowing" to get me tapping. I finally had a way to safely and creatively express my perception of this dynamic life, and it was also a way of being of service to others.

Ah, I wish for a world that gives easy access to the arts, to have dance, music, painting, sports, and nature accessible to our children, a way to express that which is unexpressed and unable to be expressed. The arts provide a safe way to integrate, release, empty, distill and transform our blues, our grievances, our knowing and un-knowing. I recall the pain in my heart in the 1980s when many of the public schools in Chicago started removing sports and music from the curriculum.

Listening and following rhythms later became my foundational form of Sound as Bodywork. I tapped the rhythms of what I was sensing. Listening and following the rhythm of peoples' bodies is key to the accuracy of sound healing.

She's Got the Nerves

I was a Highly Sensitive person and came from a town of Highly Sensitives. It was common knowledge that many inhabitants of Eldorado suffered from what was commonly called "the nerves." I'd hear whispers, "Well, you know so-and-so's got the nerves." Today it might be called anxiety or stress. And it seemed to affect almost everybody.

I always had a nerve problem. I was very sensitive, prone to depression, anger, and nervous breakdowns. Being able to see energetically from birth encouraged this. I could see the aura around people and interpret their mood state from the shape of the auric field and its colors. Sometimes there would be a scent that accompanied the mood states. Seeing in this way made a lasting imprint inside my body and affected my nervous system.

The Nerves

I come from a place where everybody had "the nerves."
Actually, it was sorta at an epidemic proportion
In the early to middle 1950s.
And it seems like I had them bad.
Grannie Ola and Verdia Rister
would sit out there on the side porch, snapping beans,
And say, "Uh huh, yup, that Vickie Ann,
She's got 'the nerves' alright.
Comes by it rightly, I'd say.
Given how her Daddy drinks," Verdia says.
Knowing what she's starting up now with Ola,
now we've got fighting words.
"Well, I never," says Grannie. "Johnny doesn't drink!"

Now you need to know.
Johnny hasn't been sober since I was born,
and Grannie lives with us, but she doesn't see.
That is how it goes. You see.
The "nerves" come in from several directions.
One of the knots of tension that gets wound up in your gut is when
"He hits the porch,"
as my Momma says about Dad's homecoming.
"Everybody act right now. He's tight."
Then the downright meanness
Of his particular kind of drunk.
"If I catch you, I'm going to kill you."

So, I run like hell, and hide myself under the bed,
pressing and flattening my body
up against the bed springs
Trying to meld my way into them
so if'n he were to look under the bed
he wouldn't be able to see me,
Just the lumpy bedsprings.
I wait there holding, my fingers and toes aching from being wrapped
around the wire springs.
I don't know how long I wait; he doesn't come.
I can hardly get unwound from the grip
As I try to quietly see if he is waiting for me.
Everything is still in the house.
Oh Lordy!
He's passed out on the couch!
Now this occurs regularly, like an army drill.
And we don't seem to ever learn,
that is just Daddy's way of greeting his family.

Then there's another form of contribution to the nerves—
the denial that any of that ever happened.
"'cause Johnnie doesn't drink."
You don't mention it,
that you were trapped melting into the bedsprings,
'cause it might make him mad; shoot, hurt his feelings.
"'cause you know, honey, he just loves you so much," my momma says.
Forgetting how just yesterday,
he had a knife and threatened to kill her,
as she runs down the road trying to reach Virginia Baggot's house.
Dad is scared of Baggot.

Then there's Grandma Berthie, my Momma's mamma, rocking,
whether it was a rocking chair or not,
She'd be rocking and biting her fingernails down to the quick,
she'd say, "bit my nails down to the quick" waiting . . . worrying . . .

29

she had "the nerves" bad, too,
like me, and I sure wanted to be like her.
She loved flowers, growing them.

What else might be the cause of "the nerves"?
Worry is a big one.
Worried can't pay the rent,
or pay down the bill at Reeder's grocer,
Worried that James (Mamma's brother)
is gonna fight with Aunt Alma (Daddy's sister)
Who is James' wife's mother –
who was my aunt and cousin . . .
You see it gets complicated,
and that is worrisome to a body, just that.
There's just no accounting for the many ways one can be
tangled up deep inside the guts with the nerves.
No wonder we can't trust what we feel or know.
The message lines are on overload.

I personally know of three nervous breakdowns
I had by the time I was 17. First one I was about 10.
Thank goodness, I was taken up into a ship,
and the folks all had white lab coats on,
and they treated me really kind,
and held my wrists and said to each other—
"Her nervous system is already polluted . . . burnt out."
And they did something that kept me going
till the next time they helped me.
Polluted, such a good word.
That's what my people called you when you were drunk,
they'd say, "He's polluted."
Fits, doesn't it?

Then there's the hypervigilance of it all . . .
Need to always know what might happen, how someone might be,

what they're thinking, or might think,
if they knew what you were thinking or doing or . . .
I mean if Daddy's having a bad day, you better act like you are, too.
You're not allowed to feel good.
It is too dangerous to get comfortable, you know,
'cause then the deep disappointment of the sky falling
becomes too much to take.
So, it is best to not feel what you feel, just know what others feel.
Keep your nervous system out there attached to each other
and to the past and the probable future wreckage,
and then you'll be fine and not cause trouble.

So now you can possibly see how "the nerves" are a hereditary disease
and should not be taken lightly . . .
even the local doctor in town knew this and
started throwing valium at you walking down the street!
This did help keep folks feeling fine.
They were fondly called "tranquilizers."
Being a Highly Sensitive person, may be a product of "the nerves"
. . . just a thought.
Running everyone's mood state
through your body, then you'd know how to respond,
as now you knew how they felt, so that's how you feel.

Awakening to a Larger Purpose

At 11 years old, I made an agreement with myself: If life did not get easier by the time I was 17, I would kill myself. I needed relief from the pain of feeling the sensations I experienced from life in general. I did not know how to protect myself. I did not know how to nourish my nervous system. I did not know how to keep my nervous system focused in my body and not constantly reaching out to others.

My family moved to Chicago. Economics and community life were changing in rural America, and many people had to migrate to the cities. I missed nature and its softness and the knowingness of earth-based

31

living. We were in much concrete among millions of people. Life did not get easier, but much harder in the vastness and diversity of city life. At 17, I had a plan to throw myself in front of an "El" train. Dying was not frightful; living was most difficult.

An inner voice, a sonic guide, which had always been with me, at this important juncture instructed: "You cannot die out of what ails you. You must learn how the emotions live within the physical body or you will be dead."

This was very depressing to one who believed the only relief was to die, and now to learn dying will not relieve this pain, and that dying is not a way out!

I was given an assignment—to learn how the emotions live within the physical body.

I now had a reason to live and was on track to learn what I needed to survive. It was the beginning of a lifelong, a life longed-for, healing. It was also the beginning of the humanistic psychology and mind–body therapies being made available here in the United States. The timing was perfect, I'm telling you!

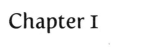

Chapter I

It's All in the Listening

"You can only listen when the mind is quiet, when there is an interval between your reaction and what is being said. There is a silence in which alone there is a comprehension which is not intellectual understanding. In that interval, there comes clarity. It is the interval that is the new brain. The new brain allows understanding and a new listening."

~ Jiddu Krishnamurti, philosopher and educator

The Issues Are in the Tissues

Please note, when I speak of the "body," I am speaking of the physical, emotional, mental, and spiritual consciousness contained in this skin and bones package we call our body. We work on the body because we can access all dimensions through the physical form. As we touch the body with sound, we can feel and see the changes that occur.

*All that has ever happened to us is recorded
in our bodies as frequencies.*

Whether engaged in self-care or as a practitioner in service to others, I need to come from a place of being empty, not an agenda of how I'm going to fix anything in those I serve. My intention is to listen, to sense from a place of not knowing. My job is to be as focused and present as possible in my listening, as I reflect an audible soundprint of what the body wants to express.

As I touch someone's magnetic field, I listen as if I am blind and reading Braille. I follow and see from my inner vision the pathways that wish to be expressed. This listening reveals a palette of pulse, rhythm, and timing; of tempo, melody, shape, form, color, and even words. These outer soundings resonate with what is familiar in that person's inner wisdom, inner teachings, and their own language.

The Formula Is Revealed

Students often want to learn techniques that will promise specific results. In Sacred Sound sessions, we do not know the formula until the body reveals it to us. Our work with sound is an emerging composition comprised of mixed elements.

The body is exquisitely intelligent and knows exactly what is needed—the timing, sequence, and tonal qualities. We are listening and trusting and following the innate wisdom of the body. We only know the formula of a session and what has occurred after the treatment is complete. The formula is being revealed during the session. It's an active trust that the body will show us what it needs and wants.

We are following the body's map. Our posture of listening is one of trusting. If we love what we want to know, it will reveal its teachings to us. Listening from love, and with love, takes time and trust and patience. We do not know beforehand what the body will reveal, because listening is an evolving formula, never a pre-planned formula. Mind wants to know ahead of time; body reveals what is in the moment. Listen to the tissue!

I do not say, "I'm going to hum here, release sounds there . . ." I come to the body willing to listen and observe, breathe and move. Together we experience what arises. We only know what different approaches were used by observing the outcome. The body unravels and unwinds in its most accurate integrity for itself.

While sounding for myself or my clients, I have found it helpful to record my perceptions in a journal in the order in which they make themselves known. I also observe how one action engaged the next.

Through keeping a journal, we start to see the sequencing of the formulas; we understand our perceptions; we see the patterns and rhythms, the characters, and subtle layers. The languages of the body are revealed, and the communication pathways are enhanced. The work becomes powerful because we start learning how the body wants to communicate with us. We develop a trust that there really is an inherent intelligence ready and willing to communicate with us. We are following the body's map.

The body is listening to see if we are listening.
Even if we are inaccurate,
the body will make it accurate.
The body is a very forgiving teacher.

All beings are aware if we are listening.
All beings are aware if we are listening with acceptance of what is.
Acceptance of what is,
is the key for transformation.

Can I be in acceptance of myself exactly as I am?
I need not be any different than who and how I am to be seen and received by grace.

Can I be in acceptance of exactly how you are?

We Sound to Get Quiet Enough to Listen

We sound the noise, the static, the ongoing conversation, the worries. We sound that which may be in the way of our listening to our audible body. The body is listening to see if we will listen. The earth is waiting to see if we will listen. The trees and plant world are waiting to see if we will listen. May we be willing to slow down enough to receive our listening.

Our work with sounding is comprised of formulas; mixtures of listening, observing, asking permission, noticing rhythms, timings, shapes, colors, breath, messages from all parts of the body, as well as all our various characters, archetypes, and ages that are encased in this garment called the body. We are asking to be in relationship and to have communication with all aspects of Self. This way of relating to ourselves is the most intimate relationship we can have.

Core essentials of the listening practice are Love and Respect.

We come to the body desiring to be in relationship with that to which we are listening. Since the mind may become impatient, we must remember to be patient—to pause and give time and space to build a new relationship with the body. Basically, slow down and develop trust. This is not a race! Trusting relationships takes time.

> "Ears are no good for this music,
> The whole presence must be open to it.
> It is a matter of vibrations."
> ~ **G.I. Gurdjieff,** philosopher and mystic

If You Love Something Enough

Respect is truly the first and foremost important ingredient for accessing trust and listening. We can get lost in our zest for healing and doing what needs to be done. In this "eager to help" mindset, our passion can move us faster than the layer at hand. It is essential to pause and remember that possibly not all parts of this being may be on the same page—not all parts of the body are eagerly awaiting our touch and sound. We wait and listen, for that which wants to be addressed will indeed bubble up to meet us. Whether we are caring for ourselves, or as a practitioner caring for others, we support the practice of listening by noticing the rhythm of our own breath and allowing it to center us.

The essential teachings of listening are an ancient system of directly cultivating relationships and communication with the mineral, plant, animal, and human world. Find your own words, but the essence is always an invitation filled with love and respect.

Body Listening Prayer

Body, I pray to be your student.
I pray to be teachable.
I come to you, my body, from a place of not knowing.
I come to you with a sincere desire
to know how to be in relationship with you.
I come wanting to know how you wish to communicate.
I'm here to learn from you.

Body, I come to you with love and respect,
How would you have me listen?
How would you have me perceive?
Body, I come to listen with all my senses.
I pause in silence and give you space to reveal your teachings.
I give thanks for the opportunity to begin this listening relationship.
I observe and am a witness, not a judge.
I enter meditative listening.

If I love something enough, it will reveal itself to me.
I come to you willing to listen.
How can I best serve you?
How can I better know you?
How would you have me be?
How would you have me listen?
What would you have me know?
Be respectful.
Give thanks.
Pause in the silence.
Listen with all your senses.

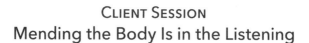

Client Session
Mending the Body Is in the Listening

This is the first of the most potent teachings of the power of listening that came in my early days of sounding bodies. It is truly humbling to know how little I knew in those days, and how much the body of sound would reveal.

In 1983, I was working out of my Chicago apartment doing Aston Massage. The manager of the apartment building, a Polish immigrant, and a survivor of a concentration camp in WW2, asked if I would be willing to give her a massage for a reduction of rent. As a single mom, I immediately replied, "Yes, thank you!"

Her trust in our relationship resulted in my working with many of her friends and family. I did only Aston massage with her, as I was still very cautious about introducing audible sound into the sessions.

For 10 years, I had been sounding clients silently, having gained permission inwardly from their soul. Many friends and folks with whom I shared mutual trust welcomed the audible sound, but there was not much support yet for sound frequency as a healing modality, even in the alternative health world. That said, during these days I used colored light bulbs at different angles on parts of the body. Color *is* sound, and I understood the colored light frequencies were the placeholders for the unexpressed sound frequencies I was sensing.

I had observed from our very first session that my client had missing toes and a frozen quality at her ankles. She was not comfortable speaking about the cause, so I respectfully did the work without probing. After some time, a trust had developed between us, and I asked whether she would mind if I made audible sounds while I was working with her.

"Go ahead," she said, "just don't stop what you are doing!"

On this day, as I began sounding and singing her body, she started to cry. Crying is not unusual when our hearts are touched, memories are stirred, and soul is acknowledged. We often cry from joy, relief, gratitude, and remembrance.

Through her tears, she exclaimed, "You're singing her song! That was what she was singing!" And then she told me this chilling tale:

We were taken to a dark cellar. So many of us packed into this cellar. We stood in water to our knees. It was so dark we couldn't see our hands in front of us. We didn't know what was to become of us. We were all terrified. Terror was moving through the water like bolts of electricity. Then a woman started singing, and she kept singing. I don't know who she was. I never could see her. You just sang her song! You sang the song she kept singing! The water calmed. The fear eased. A breath came. She saved our sanity, maybe our very lives. She sang us sane, so that we could stand and live again, as whole as possible. That's where I lost my toes. But I didn't lose my sanity or humanity.

This woman's body taught me a deep truth in that precious session. Through being willing and able to listen and make audible her body's sound frequencies, she received what she needed to mend, to heal another layer, and to digest. I will always be grateful for this dear woman. She gave me the trust and opportunity to listen and safely reveal memories embedded in her tissue.

This experience humbled me to the deep mystery and taught me: The body mends in the listening–by following the listening. Mending is not in the sounding. We do not need to put sound or anything else into a body. What is needed for expression, mending, and healing is already encoded, recorded, and imprinted within the body. We can trust that. Rest assured.

We must practice learning to read the body's language and permit its expression. We interpret from all our senses. We "act as if" it is possible to be in communication. Our journey is to recognize how the body wants to communicate with us. We become students of our bodies. We want to be in relationship with that which we desire to know, with that to which we are listening. Sounding ourselves, or our students and clients, we trust that each hears what they need to hear within the sounds, frequencies, and rhythms of our sounding.

Each of us receives and perceives what we need for our own release, healing, and integration. This potent life story and many other stories through the years taught me that Sacred Sound sessions are not about my singing skills, or my perception skills, or even about me.

We are not teaching techniques. We are teaching being in relationship. We are teaching ourselves to listen and perceive. Sessions are about the power of listening to the body and following and trusting something greater than ourselves.

Note: See Appendix 3 for more on my downloadable album, *Rest Assured: Parasympathetic Resonance*. The album invites intention to rest, to entrain, to restore and to remember how to live within the parasympathetic nervous system.

Trusting the Innate Wisdom of the Body

When we listen to what wishes and desires to be expressed, we touch the inner needs and the well of wisdom of the person we are sounding. Our intention is to access the innate wisdom of the body. As I sincerely want to listen and communicate, and truly want to be in relationship to this

40

soul, I will express what is there. I need not embellish, enhance, protect, or judge what is being expressed. What is sounded is gold for the person receiving the sounding. The body knows if it is being listened to and accepted and loved for all that it is.

Essential Tools for Listening

- Love what is.
- Respect what is.
- Appreciate and accept what is.
- Ask permission to enter and listen—each time.
- Let the body know your intention to touch, listen, and sound.
- "Act as if" it is completely natural, reasonable, and possible to have a direct relationship with the bodies of others and ourselves.

Listening is the ancient art of communication. We can be in direct communication with the life that is around us and with our bodies. Consider how our ancestors knew which plant to pick and what was its nature and remedy. We go to a plant we want to know and ask permission from the plant to learn from it. Receiving permission, we express our intention. We do the same with a human body.

We say to the plant, "I desire to know you better." We observe its color, flowers, number of petals, leaf structure, and stem. Is it round, square, fuzzy? We observe how we feel by truly being with the plant. We taste it and spit it out. Is it sour, sweet, bitter, drying to the tongue? What is its smell? Let us listen.

Like coming to know the plant we can also come to know our body. Where in my body has my attention been drawn? Interestingly, I'll start noticing my liver or my stomach or my knees. In this moment, the plant is teaching me. I am aware of my body area because the plant is communicating with me there.

The yellow flower of the dandelion brings an awareness of my liver and kidney area as I taste the bitter of its leaves and it tells me. "I am your first cleanser in the spring." Or the willow may bring my awareness to my knees or bony structure and suggest, "I can help your limbs become more resilient and flexible." These are suggestions to allow ourselves to trust our listening. The roses often teach through the sense of smell and color. The fragrance of rose fills our being with love. Wait, observe, and listen. I like to have a notepad with me, so I can jot down impressions.

I have had the privilege of living in beautiful places where one can find fields of yarrow or arnica. My herbalist teachers took us on journeys to sacred spots, and we would lie in these fields and listen with all our senses.

Even in our smaller gardens, we can sit by the plant and note what we sense. This is a lovely way to begin acknowledging we can be in communicative relationship with the plant life around us. There are many reasons we enjoy sitting with our backs resting against or hugging a tree: We receive much needed connection. Being with nature reconnects us with our own innate nature. We are developing our acuity with plants. Once we can listen to nature, we can listen to bodies more easily. We are nature.

Listening and Sounding the Soul Signatures

In the 1970s and 1980s, I sounded large circles of people. We gathered in open outdoor spaces or at conferences and retreats. With much energy and passion, I moved from one person to the next, sounding what I was then calling Soul Signatures or the Sound Prints of each person. I felt like a concert master merging with musicians in a grand orchestra.

At one of the earliest gatherings, my dear friend Kay Gardner and I listened and sounded and drummed the earth's rhythms with our hands onto the earth. A resonating energy field was created that gave us perceptible ability for listening and responding. This brought so much joy to our hearts.

This was long before sound healing became a known and respected profession. Kay was one of the few women in the sound world at that time, and was highly respected as an accomplished musician and well-known recording artist. She composed one of the first recordings of the *chakras*, the body's energy centers, and drawings of chakras were included in her album.

Since Soul Signatures and Sound Prints flowed in strings of rhythmic syllables, people often asked what language I was sounding. And many told me I was speaking Spanish, Zuni, Hopi, Mongolian, Hebrew, and Slavic dialects. Everyone heard something different! I was sounding or acknowledging their soul.

For me, the teaching revealed that everyone heard or interpreted something different. My interpretation was that they heard what their soul needed to have revealed or have digested. It was becoming more evident that sounding was about listening, and others would hear what they needed to hear. Not just my listening but the listeners' listening. The rhythms of the sounding take on a familiar cadence of language that resonates within the person receiving the sounding. Each hears what they need to hear or remember. Our focus with sounding is matching a resonance that wishes to be expressed.

Keys to Perception

We all perceive in different ways. We may perceive through words, colors, sound, felt sense, shapes, and images. When we listen, we are inquiring as to what the body wishes to reveal.

The body is always communicating with you. What is your form of listening? What is your preferred way of perceiving? You may have many diverse forms. Here are a few examples of how a body may communicate with you. Simply observe.

- Do you perceive colors around an area?
- Do you sense a discomfort in the lower back or feel nausea in the stomach?
- Do you perceive a sound, hear a hum, a rhythm, a laugh, a cry?
- Does the tissue look shiny?
- Is there a lot of heat in an area directly on the body or a few inches above the area of attention?
- Do you notice a scent?
- A taste in your mouth?
- Has breathing changed?
- Does the area appear shortened, perhaps due to tension in the area?
- Does it appear out of proportion to another area above or below?

- Do you see an image?
- Does the auric field, or their energy field, have your attention?
- What else calls to your attention?

Wake up to your possibilities of listening. Listen from the place of "not knowing," the beginner's mind. Simply notice.

EXERCISE
Perception

- Close your eyes, and become quiet and still. Purposely tune in by focusing your attention on grounding–plugging in, being present and respectful. "Being where your feet are."
- Visualize your whole body in the form of an ear, from the top of your head to your toes.
- Take on the shape of an ear.
- Allow your body's "felt sense" (See *Focusing* by Eugene Gendlin, 1982) to be an antenna that can perceive frequency and vibration from every crevice and molecule of your physical form. (Listening in this way is like looking for the light switch in a dark room.)
- Slowly, gently, you feel your way around the field.
- Be mindful. There is no need to reach out to listen; the direction is always inward.
- You may ask a question to guide your listening or wait to see if your body wants to give you a message unasked.
- Allow the body to reveal what it wishes to communicate.

Physicality of Codependency

Talking about listening, and the teachings that come from listening, reminds me of the oak tree that gave me a life-long teaching that keeps informing me that the most important thing I can do is to mend and heal my nervous system daily.

A long time ago, I was walking along the Baden Sea, a body of water that separates Switzerland and Germany to the north. It was a sparkling, warm, sunny, late autumn day. I only had a few days left of my visit before returning home to the US. My trip had been especially successful and fulfilling. The classes had gone well; no upsets with students or housing situations. I was feeling exceedingly fortunate and happy for this fortuitous time.

This was my day off, and I was in the country for a walk to relax and relish this moment. Just prior to starting my walk, I checked my email and read a message about a teacher from three decades earlier who became a friend of mine, a teacher I still admire. We often exchange written cards.

As I walked along, I found myself thinking about many years past. Suddenly, I started feeling regret and shame that I hadn't gotten my degree in Anthropology! And I hadn't stayed here and hadn't gone there, and if only I had done this instead of that. You get my drift?

In a matter of minutes, I was thousands of miles away, and 30 years into the past and 30 years into the future, with many people and many conversations and configurations. I was in stories of regret of the wreckage of my past and fearful of the wreckage of my future.

I could see clearly in those moments with my inner sight. My nervous system was like fat spaghetti noodles living outside my body and reaching to other people and places from all directions. I was plugged into infinite scenarios both real and imagined.

All this happened within a few moments and seemingly involuntarily—a spontaneous explosion coming out of a "joyful and success" space in time. I have great respect for the many layers of memory and the timings for the memories to be revealed for another teaching and healing.

Within moments, my beautiful, successful, abundant life had evaporated into a dissatisfying, painful, hopeless situation. I was stopped in my tracks. I noticed that I was standing next to a plowed field of lumps of hardened earth and across this field stood a big oak tree. I heard it calling to me, *Come. Are you ready for your next teaching?* In that instant, I entered a dimension that was beyond and separate from that of the people walking on the trail.

It was a long trudge across this hardened, turned-over earth, especially since I was mentally suffering from my inner lamenting. I looked down at my brand-new pair of red leather shoes that I dearly loved! They were being ruined, but I no longer cared. My life sucked, and I needed help!

As I got nearer, I could see a willow and a birch tree standing with the oak. Reaching the oak tree, I fell on my knees at its rooted feet and burst out crying. I told the oak how tired I was after all these years of trainings and self-work, meditations, and spiritual disciplines. I told the great oak that I was such a mess, and I just wanted to stop this misery!

"I need help!" I was crying and talking out loud. To this day, I have no idea if anyone saw or heard me; it never crossed my mind.

I vulnerably confessed to the oak tree as I lay there in an altered state. The oak tree gave a felt sense of a "nod" and bent toward the willow and birch trees, as if the trio were conferring with each other. The oak then came back to me, and in a commanding manner communicated:

"You could do what we do."

I jumped at this. "Yes, yes. What is that?"

The oak said, "We mind our own business!"

At the instant that I received this teaching from the trees, all the strands of my nervous system snaked rapidly back into my body, very much like the cord in my vacuum cleaner recoils when I move the handle. All those strands of nervous system that were "out there," 30 years ago, 30 years in the future, and 3,000 miles away; all the many stories of family, students, lovers, events that were held together by my strung-out nervous system strands. Yes, "strung out" is a good term! My system responded as if a great magnetic force had created a unified field inside my body.

The experience laid me out flat on the ground for some time, as my body received a rush of vitality and energy-filled breath. I rested there in a timeless state of being. If people noticed me, they had no impulse to check on me or interfere. I'm so grateful. I was protected from the moment this transmission began. I lost all sense of time, and I know for several minutes or an hour I could not move.

The Teachings of the Trees

The trees were instructing me telepathically, making it possible for me to feel myself as a whole embodied soul. This was a physical nervous system retrieval that allowed me to see and feel the visceral embodiment of my own nervous system.

Now, I fully understood the oak tree's command.
Minding my own business meant keeping my nervous
system in my own body so it could mend.

I knew in that moment that stretching my nervous system out like an antenna to feel what others are thinking, feeling, and experiencing in their bodies was my physicality of codependency. The nervous system does not know real or imagined, good or bad news; it just knows news.

When we unplug from our Source and plug into others, our own circuits can become burnt out, and we start minding the business of others instead of our own business.

Since childhood, I'd used my own vitality and my physical nervous system to listen, to plug into others, and to move through the world; this was the only way I knew how to sense the inner and outer workings of my surroundings.

The blessed Oak, Willow, and Birch Trees transmitted two
transformational teachings: Do not use my physical nervous system to
connect with others. Do not use my own physical vitality to listen.

The trees also gifted me a powerful felt sense of knowing when I was using my nervous system to extend beyond the boundaries of my own core body into others, and when I was resting in my own body and receiving. Now the deep work of reeducating my neurological system began.

How to Mind My Own Business

How could I stay resting in myself and connect with people and life around me? I knew innately that digesting the experience of these sacred instructions from the trees would be a full-time training for me. I did not have verbal or a cognitive frame of reference with which to create new neural pathways of listening and attending to myself and others.

I began a daily practice of noticing when my nervous system extended outside my core—a long, familiar, habitual neurological pathway since childhood. Every few minutes, I had to consciously interrupt and choose to bring my nervous system back home and listen from my core being. I also started using my Hum resonance, audibly and silently, to call it back home (discussed in depth in chapter 2). This daily self-care has continued and helps ensure that I stay connected and rested within myself. I have called this practice "Minding My Own Business," as the trees taught, and it makes sense.

My business is taking care of my nervous system, taking care of my health, and staying out of the way of others. If I mind my own business, my nervous system, I need not mind the business of others.

While Humming, I find it helpful and comforting, touching the front of my body, the center core, from the throat to the pubic bone. Following my frontal spine and gently touching the front of my torso while Humming, I have the intention of calling my nervous system back home to my body. I do this exercise slowly, allowing time to feel myself coming home. We come home, one fascia strand at a time.

Overview of the Oak Tree's Sacred Teachings

- Take responsibility for knowing what is mine and what belongs to others.
- Honor myself fully by taking care of my own needs.
- If in any way, I am hurting myself while serving others, the serving is an illusion.

I am reframing what being a healer means. The lineage and mythology of being a healer has long been one of sacrifice. If I am wearing myself thin, I am not truly being of service to myself or others, and the essential integrity of my being is sacrificed by this codependency. What is the new framing?

If one decides they want to be a healer, they have made an agreement to heal themselves.

Years ago, I called the physical/emotional feeling of being strung out "psychic codependence." I did not know how to stay out of other people's business. But I didn't really know how to cease doing this, let alone teach others. I hadn't seen the physicality of codependency so directly until the trees revealed to me energetically what I was unable to grasp mentally. I only knew to recognize it and to cut the cords when the circuitry got overloaded.

I did not know the immense possibilities of symptoms that resulted from this type of codependent nervous system connection. This was, and is, so huge I could barely grasp it. I sat with those Tree Teachings and let them penetrate to my very soul and to my cells. I knew I was being instructed in a profound way—so visceral, so ethereal, so real, and so nebulous, all at the same time.

Through the instructions relayed by the oak tree I was shown the physicality of my own codependency and my sovereignty. Simultaneously, I saw the responsibility of minding my own business as an honoring of self, a privilege, a human right of embodiment, an emotional maturity. I take care of myself and others by living from the wisdom of my own nervous system.

The trees showed me that my neural pathways were well versed in literally reaching out to others—in my loving, in my worrying, in my jealousies, in my caring, in my healing, in my judgments, in all my relationships. Restoring the nervous system is foundational to all aspects of health. May I come home to my own body.

Chapter 2

The Power of the Hum

The Hum of Mama's Voice

My mother had a voice like syrup . . . Just saying hello.
A soothing, soothing voice.
Standing by the kitchen table or at the kitchen door,
I can see her so plainly . . .
She would start swaying and clapping the side of her leg,
Finding . . . listening . . .
to the rhythm of the song that was going to come.
And she'd start moving.
"Ummmmmm . . . the sun's gonna shine on my back door someday."
I just remember the musicians saying,
"It's hard to follow Verbel, as you never know what she's going to do."
Mama was following the wave of the feeling
that was coming through her, not the notation of the music chart.
When I was in her womb, she'd say,
"I prayed you would have a voice. I prayed you would be strong,
I prayed you would not have my life."
What an unconditional love prayer.
Thank you, Mama.

My mother wanted me to have my own voice, the freedom to speak my truth. However, that got me a lot of sore ankles. She would kick me under the table, as I always wanted to speak up and say what I thought or saw. Women and girl children were really to be seen and not heard. They were not to have voices. Mama was always saying, "Be quiet. Don't stir up stuff!" She was trying to keep both of us safe. In my rebellious, righteous youth, I thought it was my job to express the truth.

There were many profound women in my life, and my mother was one of them. I could always find her because she always had a hum going on. Whether she was scrubbing the sinks or hanging out clothes—follow the hum, find Mom. I did not reflect for several decades on the fact that my mother was innately keeping a sound vibration going in her body. Her life was most challenging, filled with much fear about the unknowable, explosive actions of others most anytime during the day. Living with daily terror of what might occur any moment would, and could, easily create a rigid, frozen body.

I believe from my deepest knowing that Mama's innate wisdom of keeping frequency resonance alive in her body with her singing and humming sustained a resiliency that allowed her to retain a loving dignity within herself and toward others. I do believe that Mama's humming was keeping me resilient as well.

Keeping a resonance in our bodies, we are being of service to those in our environments and to ourselves. Our resonance creates an aliveness in our beings—if I have movement going on in my body, it is going to affect those in my environment.

We entrain so easily. We energetically broadcast whatever is going on. If I am fearful, stressed, or impatient, I am communicating that without saying any words aloud. Humming is a way I can help myself during times of feeling fear. When I take my own Hum as a mantra to keep myself liquid, I become a helpful member of society, instead of adding confusion and fear to an overladen situation.

Let me bring the Hum into me. Let me be a more neutral being. The Tibetan monks have been teaching us for decades that we chant to become silent. The Hum has always been the foundation of Sacred Sound Works. The magic and beauty of the Hum is that it soothes, clears, and massages our inner terrain.

The Valuable Benefits of Humming

- Humming begins any sound work—it is an opening, a doorway.
- Humming is soothing to the nervous system—it is our innate de-stressor.
- Humming keeps us present, neutral, and sustains our dynamic nature.
- Humming is nutrition—it is a nourishing food, like vitamin B.
- Humming is a protective shield—it is our resonant boundary.
- Humming increases our core magnetism, attracting ourselves back home.
- Humming is our Soul Retrieval song.
- Humming is integrating—it assimilates all our sound work.
- Hum as a loving acceptance of self.

Keys to Accessing the Humming Voice

"The wave we think of as sound actually passes more easily and swiftly through the liquids and solids of the body as a whole than it does through air to reach the ear as sound."

~ Julie Henderson, model

Our physical body is a terrain of approximately 70 percent liquid. The Hum vibration creates a wavelike motion in our liquidity that creates a rearrangement of our liquid homeostasis. The Hum acts as a pulsation, which ignites the fire that sets up a wave movement throughout our body. It gently and lovingly awakens and enlivens our dynamic nature.

Key No. 1:
We use the speaking voice, not the singing voice

I teach all Sacred Sound principles through our speaking voice. As singers, we are trained to vocalize the right pitch, rhythm, and tone of the scored composition. Our speaking voice is literally how we commonly talk with someone, and how we speak our name when introduced. We are not trying to "sound" a certain way. The speaking voice untouched and unmodified reveals how we really are physically and emotionally.

Key No. 2:
Our voice is directed inward

With this practice, we are injecting our Hum, instead of projecting it. Our intention is to bring this sound resonance inside the body. Typically, when we sing, teach, or converse we are projecting our sound outward into the room toward the audience. With our speaking voice, we are swallowing our sound inwardly, to feel the Hum flow inside our bodies. Practice and intention are essential to reframe and retrain this inward direction of sound. By projecting sound in, not out, we are "informing" our body with our sound.

Key No. 3:
The Hum begins our sound work

It is a doorway. Humming sets the stage for our foundational work. It sets up the neutral canvas and platform for our listening, providing an entry into this inner mystery. The Hum creates a field of attention for the many characters, cells, and systems inside the body; it is a signal that work is beginning. This ensures that all these aspects of self are safe and secure. The Hum awakens memory of cohesive purpose in the tissue, creating an internal opportunity to experience coherence.

Key No. 4:
Scanning ourselves is essential

Before we do any sounding, I recommend taking a scan of ourselves. Where are we physically, emotionally, psychologically, spiritually in this moment? We want to see how sound works in our body, to experience what occurs. I suggest you take a walk around your room or outside. Notice where the weight is in your feet? Is it more to the outside, more at your heel? Notice how you are feeling emotionally. What are your thoughts about? Is there any place in your body that is talking to you? You are not focusing on what is right or wrong; you are simply noticing *where* you are and *how* you are today!

This is an essential teaching to carry out before and after our sounding practices! We observe. Our body is our laboratory. You want to make a note on how you are feeling before and after you sound. Basically, you will be discovering evidence of the power of Humming, the power of your voice. If you don't scan before, you will not have a point of reference. Before I work with people, I always have them scan their physical, emotional, and psychological body. When we end the session, I then have them re-scan and note any changes. By so doing they personally witness how the power of sound has affected their well-being.

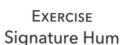

EXERCISE
Signature Hum

Our purpose is to be with our entire body as a resonance chamber. Each time we do this Signature Hum Exercise and the Soothing Hum Exercise that follows it, we are saying hello to all parts of our self, and we will naturally notice something new in every practice. I offer these exercises to help you establish awareness that your body is a resonant system. **Note:** Vickie's YouTube Hum series can be found at www.youtube/lany9lyni8o.

- Sit or stand comfortably.
- Speak your name aloud in a natural tone.
- Let your name spiral and curve inside your mouth, as if you have placed your name into a blender.
- Let the sound blend and turn into a tone, a Hum; you are swallowing your sound to direct it inward.
- This internal tone is your own Signature Hum.
- Let yourself Hummm, Hummm, Hummm for 10–30 seconds . . . breathing gently, never forcing inhalation and exhalation. When your natural exhale is complete, relax, inhale, and begin again.

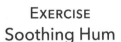

EXERCISE
Soothing Hum

- Allow your hands to touch and shape your head as you Hum.
- Be with yourself fully so that you can feel the resonance in your head. This is the easiest place to recognize resonance.
- Let your hands touch and shape your neck as you continue your Hum.
- Listen to your resonant body as you breathe and feel sensations.
- Always remember to **pause** and **notice** what you are feeling and where.
- Bring your awareness and your hands onto your chest cavity, the home of the lungs and the heart center.
- *Hummm, Hummm, Hummm.*
- **Rest, pause, breathe**, and **notice** how this feels to you.
- Continue your Hum exploration into your solar plexus, abdomen, and lower back, remembering at each location to **pause** and **notice** any sensations.
- Now attend to your limbs in the same way.

Acceptance of What Is—The Key to Transformation

My voice is shaped and influenced by my environment, inner as well as outer. The quality of my voice is affected by how much sleep I have had, what I have eaten, who I am with, my location, my body's stiffness or flexibility, a task I am doing. I don't "try" to make a "right" pitch when I speak or yawn or sigh; "what is" shapes the spontaneous sound that flows out of me.

It is the same with the Hum. I am not trying to make the right pitch. My Humming voice is spontaneous, audibly matching "what is" now. Sounding the Hum, I am being with my body, communicating to the many aspects of myself that I am in acceptance of what is, of how I am now. I only want to know myself more authentically as I am at this moment—in full acceptance. The message I am giving to myself is this:

I do not need to be any different than I am.
I do not need to change to be received, loved, or accepted.

Being in acceptance allows a resting to arise in me—a resting in my gut, in my nervous system. This resting encourages resiliency and cooperation amongst all my many parts. Through being accepted, what needs or wants to be changed and rearranged is now more available to suggestion and a restored integrity.

Sounding is not doing, not working hard, not sonically tearing through the pathways or the tissues. My body is fluid—it changes as I change. My sound changes as my inner and outer environment changes. My Hum is spontaneous. Its natural voice will be different tomorrow than it was yesterday, and different two hours from now. As the saying goes, "You cannot step in the same river twice." My body is a river.

The Hum Soothes and Reduces Stress

Humming can help neutralize some of the physical and emotional effects from a variety of situations that create coagulation of our liquid terrain: basic fatigue from a day's activities, stressful lifestyles, too much computer or television time, airplane travel, side effects related to trauma. These frequencies and situations create clusters in our molecular structure. When we are stressed, the molecules in our body stick together, jumbled like a beaver's dam. The body has lost its liquidity; there is no longer flow.

Molecules with Stress   Molecules with Sound

Go with the Flow!

Stressed molecules bunched together in the physical terrain constrict our circulation and impede flow in our liquid system. This molecular stress is felt as physical tension that, in turn, creates emotional and mental impatience in our system and musculature. The mind says: *I do not have enough room; I do not have enough time.*

As we Hum, our inner terrain softens and returns to its more dynamic rhythmic nature. We can experience longer durations of motion in our liquid system. As we Hum, we are "going with the flow," which literally creates more room for ourselves, more time, more patience, more openness. Sounding changes our perception and adjusts our attitudes.

Physical Benefits of Humming

As we Hum, the vibration and resonance of this sounding sets a coherent wave in motion throughout our body. A rearrangement of our homeostasis begins. We use intention with sound to address the nervous system.

The *Hum* and *Shhh* sounds soothe the nervous system and the superficial musculature. These sounds help hydrate the entire connective tissue layer. The Hum starts preparing the body to receive the work needed. It softens and creates a relaxing and restful experience. It is a calming tool at any time.

One of the most health-giving properties of the Hum is that it creates and sustains a flow of inner movement. When my being sustains dynamic movement, I am less prone to stressors. The Hum frequency strengthens my field, so the emotions and changing mood states of other people are less likely to set up residence in my body. How easy it is for us to pick up what is not ours—if there is movement, stress can move through us, in and out.

How do I get present? The Hum brings us into presence very quickly and easily. We find what is ours each day by doing our Signature Hum exercise. We fill ourselves up with our own resonance, that which is ours. The more my frequency magnetism increases, the more what is not mine cannot stick in my system. I have less Velcro!

> "Leave your front door and your back door open.
> Allow your thoughts to come and go.
> Just don't serve them tea."
> ~ **Shunryu Suzuki**, Soto Zen monk and teacher

The Hum as Resonance Protection

In my youth, I lacked the knowledge of how to keep my nervous system inside my own body. As a result, I experienced other people's mood states of depression, anger, fear, and sadness as if they were my own. This locked my sympathetic nervous system into a stress syndrome that also taxed my adrenals. Our language reflects symptoms of stress: "A tiger is on my tail," "I need to hurry," "There is never enough time," "Life is not safe," "I don't know who to trust," "I can't trust myself." My body was communicating with me early on, but I didn't know how to resonate with its wisdom.

When I started learning techniques to protect myself, I tried to control the energies outside myself by using various images and affirmations to construct shields of protection around me. Sound familiar? However, this created a fixed, static, holding posture in my body. Where there is stress and tension in the body, the lactic acid creates a boundary of stagnation that restricts fluid movement. Anything floating "down the river" gets caught in the beaver's dam of stagnant energy. As a result, like that beaver's dam, my shields of protection attracted to me exactly what I feared.

Using my Humming to create a protective field of harmonic resonance inside me calmed my nervous system and naturally created a protective field of harmonic resonance around me. This was the first major teaching I received from the Hum!

I still encountered the mood states of others on the city blocks—a psychotic one there, a depressive one here—but I didn't have to defend myself against these vibrations. My coherence was clear and strong enough that the frequencies of other people could be acknowledged without having them run through my body. Contrary to my previous belief system of protection, I did not have to wear an imagined fixed shield after that.

The Hum activated and enlivened the protective shield of my own vibrational coherency. I had less Velcro, less got attached within my field. Sound changes form, rearranges form, and creates form.

EXERCISE
The Hum as Resonance Protection

- Do your Signature Hum as previously taught.
- This time, as you continue to Hum, let your arms stretch and move out gently in your surrounding field and encircle your body.
- With your hands and with your Hum, you are touching your electromagnetic field, the energy body that surrounds your physical form.
- Notice how the Hum creates a dynamic vibration inside and around your physical form.
- Activate and enliven this protective shield of your own personal vibrational coherence every day, as often as you like.
- Notice how the Hum increases your magnetic field; as the Hum becomes more potent, it becomes a protector and ally.

The Hum as Healer

During a traumatic experience of any kind—drama in our relationships, abuse, bad news, strong emotions, a painful diagnosis, a car accident, and so on—we often leave our body emotionally. It is simply a knee-jerk response, like an involuntary muscle spasm. *I want to escape this reality. I am scared, I am leaving.* Parts of us fragment, splinter off, and for many reasons, known or unknown, we become detached from our vital resource, what I call Source.

I Pause, I Breathe

I love myself enough to stop for a few moments
and "plug into" the earth
and ask to be received.
We surrender to the earth
outside ourselves and inside.
We listen and see what bubbles up
to help us remember to come back.
Please bring all of me back.
I forgot, I got scared, I am worried,
I don't know what to do.

This fragmenting happens in most traumatic events. Often, we do not know this has happened, but the imprints of trauma are recorded in the body. The physical body posture is influenced and shaped from the stress of trauma; often a frozen quality to the movement arises. The paralysis of fear is really a physical experience. My brain wants to fix it, but can't function correctly, because of a frozen quality within my physiology.

When in trauma, Humming can begin to melt fear and the frozen qualities in the body. Hum out loud or silently for yourself or for someone else. Humming keeps the energy flowing so the nervous system doesn't freeze up. Humming increases our magnetism, enabling us to vibrationally entrain, or call, that which is ours back home.

The more home I am, the more present I become. When we are home, in our body, we can receive what we need: the healing frequencies that support our wellbeing. This use of the Hum is a form of soul retrieval work. Let us retrieve those parts of self, known and unknown, and bring them back home.

I encourage you to give Humming your patience and practice over time. Lying in bed or in a quiet reflective state, notice when you find yourself remembering an earlier incident, a love affair that went sour, a car accident that still haunts you, an uncomfortable place you still travel to in your thoughts, even after much inner work. Let your Hum begin. Let your Hum soothe and relax your thinking.

In these quiet times, ask yourself: *Is there a part of me that is left there? Is there a strand or part that is ready to be restored and rewoven in the fabric of my bodily pattern? I only ask for what is ready to be revealed.*

Remember we do not dig or work hard. We respect the timing of healing, while remembering that it may not be the timing we desire. Our Humming engages our essential wisdom to heal and restore self. The Hum is a compassionate self-care tool used to visit with our deeper self at any time. Humming as a self-healing practice becomes a habit.

Energetic Feng Shui

Before I leave a workshop or any social gathering, I listen and ask to bring all of me home. It is a very quiet, inner request. No one ever needs to know. I just ask for all of me to come home. Like my coat and scarf, I gather myself with my inner silent Hum. In my excitement about events or conversations and experiences that took place, I may have left some part of myself in the environment I am leaving.

I teach my students to do this self-care before they leave my seminars. Often, we have traveled through many galaxies and felt many sensations. When we leave this cocoon of safety, we may feel spaced and vulnerable as we enter the world of cars, trams, airports.

We must take a few moments before we leave and "walk around" the areas we have traveled. We scan the conversations we've had and the work we were involved in and reclaim any parts of self and frequency that may have fragmented. We Hum silently and ask them to please come home. We walk about and silently or audibly Hum to bring that which is ours back home to our body.

My magnetism of frequency attracts that which is mine back into my body as I sound the Silent Hum. I call this the "energetics of feng shui." *May I be responsible for my own energy.* I feel this is an essential self-care exercise of compassion and reverence for the sensitive beings we all are.

Also, we make good guests, as we do not leave energetics that belong with us for someone else to deal with!

The longer you work with your Hum, the more your voice will teach you of its powerful possibilities. The longer and more often you Hum, the more potent it becomes. We want our body to resonate with our inherent frequencies so that we can communicate and transmit the frequency of Hum with or without the conscious need to make the sound. This frequency communicates to all other frequencies. It creates a communication of trust and rest. As you practice, notice how your frequency changes or rearranges your perceptions.

When working with clients who are very upset, fearful, anxious, and unable to relax or be present, teach them to activate their Signature Hum. Hum along with them to support creating a sympathetic resonance and an entrainment.

This also allows clients to feel safe, not on the spot, as they are not alone with their sounding. Assisting others in using their voice for self-care empowers them. They now have a way to pause, relax, and allow a new perspective to arise. Over and over, I have experienced this. Sound works faster than any mode I know.

Hum as Meditation

In India, people tell a story about the elephant. Its keeper knows that walking the elephant through the market on festival days can be disruptive. The elephant and his trunk can be like a tornado roaring through the vendors' shops, grabbing bananas, knocking down displays, creating havoc and stress for all. The keeper has learned to give the elephant a wand to hold in its trunk, giving the trunk a focus and purpose. The elephant now has a job: to hold the wand.

People often say that they cannot meditate because they cannot quiet their minds. Ancient teachings were designed to give the mind a "wand"– a prayer, a mantra, a focus. When occupied with a focus, the mind has a job, a purpose. In turn, our mind will not interrupt our daily living with the worry and fearful thinking that leads to stress and feelings of insecurity. Mantras have been used for thousands of years, in nearly all cultures, as a kind of a prayer to occupy the mind. A common chant is *OM*. Make this sound and you'll notice that nearly half of the *OM* is a Hum. Humming silently or aloud provides a simple, powerful, meditative focus for our mind.

The Wonderful Wand of Gratitude

Our minds need a focus, a wand to hold.
Our mind needs a prayer of gratitude daily.
A wand of gratitude provides the opportunity to awaken.
Humming soothes the body, emotions, and mind.
as we focus on the wonderful wand of gratitude.

Trust and Not Knowing

We are sounding without expectation of outcome. This is a spiritual teaching: sound as our teacher. Can we trust that there is a power greater than our "knowing," and are we willing to trust and surrender to something greater than our "knowing"?

We never know what we are going to sound. We step into the liquid. We come from a place of being curious. We come from a place of not knowing. Our Hum is a doorway, an entry into this inner mystery school. As we Hum, our body will start revealing and asking for other sounds and combinations. We begin the practice with our Hum, as it allows us to stay authentic to ourselves.

The longer you work with the Hum, the more your voice will teach you the possibilities of its power. The longer and more often we make this sound, the more potent it becomes. That is why the Hum begins and closes our daily sound practices.

May these teachings speak to you and assist your discovery of sound frequency as a sacred, spiritual body of work. The Hum has many teachings and more to come, this one can trust.

Rest Assured

Quietly rest, my Beloved.
So much does the outer world disrupt you,
So much is confusion in that world,
That more than all else,
You need a time for simple resting in My Love,
And a drinking in of my Peace.

Come close that I may enfold you.
Rest, Rest Assured.
Put aside all thought of confusion and distress
And allow My divine plan to flow through you and all your affairs.

So, step aside for a few moments
From that world so full of distress,
And resting in my presence
You shall be able to fulfill your destiny
And the service you were meant to do.

Note: See Appendix 3 for more information on my downloadable album *Rest Assured: Parasympathetic Resonance.* The album invites intention to rest, to entrain, to restore, and to remember how to live within the parasympathetic nervous system.

Chapter 3

Vocabulary of Sounds

Sounding is a way to dissolve undigested material, matter that has become embedded in the tissue. The sounding language can "chew up" stuck, sticky matter that has become hardened, dense, flat, or numb. Any number of possibilities can take place within our physiology to create a lack of responsive resonance in the muscular/fascia system. This denser matter can restrict the physical, three-dimensional volume capacity of our body.

Our sound language can dissolve, stimulate, and soothe the often-times frozen or seemingly unresponsive matter. Our being has the inherent wisdom to receive what is needed to balance and restore health and regeneration within the muscular/fascia system. Remember, sound has nutritional components.

I am asking you to use your body as your laboratory, your teacher, and to suggest this experimentation to your clients and students.

The Wisdom of Vowels

The power of the vowels started healing, mending, and melting the frozenness in my entire bodily system. The result of excess sensitivity, of perceiving more than I was capable of expressing, affected my expression center, the throat. My throat was nearly paralyzed (frozen); the aperture became very narrowed so that when I spoke, people could barely hear me. This frozenness developed over time from my youth.

In my private practice I was sounding silently, as my voice was nearly closed. I would ask permission from the person's soul to silently sound their body and visualize the sound as it moved through their body. This helped me develop a strong mental capacity to focus, listen, observe, and remain present with what the client's body revealed.

Elias DeMohan, who started the first sound school in the US in 1958, was the only person I knew who was working with sound. He seemed to understand what I perceived and encouraged me in this pursuit. Elias directed me to the vowels and his form of teaching them with color and emotional qualities.

I could barely make the sounds, but with Elias's instruction of visualization, intention, and gently shaping the vowels while visualizing their shape inside my body, the vibration and frequency started melting and dissolving my frozen throat.

I did not try to sonically stretch or tear tissue or attempt to break up the crystallization in my throat. I simply allowed my sounding to match the shape, rhythm, and color quality of what was available in my body. Sound frequency via the vowels was teaching me the principle of matching what is available, respecting and accepting the restriction— being present and respectful to what is, being willing to be in my own body laboratory and inquire as to what was the size of this frozen narrow aperture? It was thin, like the tiniest penny whistle. Sounds coming out of me were merely tiny squeaks.

With clear intention, I practiced noticing and matching the emotional and color qualities of each vowel from Elias's system. For example, the color for the vowel *Ah* is yellow. The positive emotional qualities of yellow are creativity and open-mindedness. The negative emotional qualities are too much analysis and criticism. We cannot have one without the other. Accept and allow it all.

As the vowels touched and massaged the narrow aperture of my throat, it softened and became larger, more open. My intention was to match and massage the shape I was sounding, not try to change it. The vowels plus intention and color were lubricating the tissue membranes.

We know that our bodies are 70–80 percent liquid, and that sounding dissolves constrictions, congestions, and crystallizations within our fluid system. As I sounded and visualized color and matched the shape, the constrictions started softening and dissolving. Through the power of sounding vowels, I directly experienced the healing power of matching and shaping the body's restorative ability to reclaim my voice.

I invite you to give yourself the time and opportunity to explore sound frequency in your body laboratory. Have your own direct experiences, so that these teachings become more than a mental theory. The vowels are in most of our languages, and they have always been regarded as sacred resonance vibrations.

Exercise
Vowel Shaping

In our explorations, we allow the vowel sounds to shape themselves inside our liquid, malleable terrain, our interior space.

The healing power of the vowel is in both the sound *and* its shaping.

- Let the vowel sounds shape themselves interiorly—in your mouth, inside your voice box, your neck, the back of your head, even your belly.
- Be with wherever the shaping wants to go.
- Notice how the vowels can shape you.
- What is the sensation or effect of this shaping?
- Imagine a vowel inside your body, expanding to fill your entire body.
- Notice how that shaping feels as you sound the vowel.
- Imagine your body as a liquid laboratory.
- Take each of the vowels into your liquid laboratory and experiment. Discover the action of their shape on your inner terrain. Remember you are liquid.
- Let the vowels take their shape inside you.

The Sound Palette—The Vocabulary of Sounds

The body likes and needs a variety of rhythms to address its many systems. Enjoy your exploration of your sound palette. Here are some sounds that have come to me and many others through the years. Jump in and see what sounds want to come to you. You may want to start here and allow them to awaken you to other sounds and their specific meanings and usages. What sounding does is help you awaken forgotten or frozen memories or deeper knowings. We are sounding to remember what we have forgotten. We are sounding to dissolve that which is in the way of what we know.

E Sound

Used as part of a formula, the *E* sound can break up emotional congestion in many parts of the body. It is especially helpful when working in the solar plexus area, which is designated by mystery schools as the body's emotional brain center. I have found the *E* sound is very helpful for clearing the head centers, especially when bringing the tongue upward as you sound nasally, toward the pineal and pituitary areas inside the brain.

HA HA HA Sounds

Our ancient medicines have always known the need to activate the vital organs in the solar plexus area. Eastern martial arts practitioners have used loud sound combinations for centuries. For instance, *HA HA HA* has been a sound used to break up congestion in the solar plexus and to strengthen *chi*, or life force. I think our living organs appreciate being noticed and addressed with the refreshing internal massage sound provides. I encourage you to explore combinations of vowels and consonants for your own sound self-care.

Shhh Sounds

Shhh is an ancient sound in all cultures and languages, and seemingly the universal sound for soothing. *Shush, shhh* . . . it's all right. *Shhhhhhh* . . . rest, be quiet, go to sleep. You're alright. *Shush, shuuu, shaah.*

Shhh is also one of the more powerful sounds as bodywork. The *shhhh, shhh* sound softens the superficial tissue, the top layer. *Shhhh, shhh* relaxes the nervous system and assists the body in becoming more liquid. This very beneficial sound can gently reveal a layer of fear or trauma stored within a body. I have done complete sessions with only the *shhh* sound and variations of its rhythms. The *shhh* sound has also taught me that when a completion of a layer of work is done, the *shhh* sound is administered with a long, drawn-out breath.

CLIENT SESSION
Soothing Trauma

Years ago, while teaching in Mexico, I worked with a young man who had been kidnapped and eventually returned to his family. His being was so very traumatized that his body was a frozen system. I gave him several sessions, all consisting of softly sounded *shhh* and Hum. These sounds were caressing and comforting for him, as they would be for a wounded child. I taught him to gently touch his body while Humming softly to himself and sounding *shhh, shhh, shhh*. Using this simple practice, the young man understood how easily he could care for himself when he couldn't sleep or when he awakened from fearful dreams, or anytime he felt nervous and afraid. I invite you to do the same. See how this feels for you.

Aerobic Sounds—
Sounding and Emptying the Inner Noise

Aerobic sounds are a compilation of vowels and consonants, sounds and gibberish noise. They are fast moving, stimulating rhythms, and staccato breath sounds. We vocalize infinite possibilities of unpredictable sounds, in any combinations and rhythms. We just let ourselves make sounds. *AH AH EH EH HO HO GRRRR.* These fast, rhythmic, aerobic sounds act as an emptying exercise that brings great release and begins the quieting. We give sound expression to our noise, our inner noisy conversation. We use fast-moving aerobic sounds as tools to restore our body to a more liquid state.

Our focus is to:

- release holding patterns in our breath
- promote movement in our systems
- empty "stuckness" physically, emotionally, and psychologically
- aid our circulation and stimulate our immune systems
- break up crystallization and dissolve congestion
- sound and empty that which is not ours to store
- get quiet.

The fast rhythms are often used to help us wake up and remember to be willing—willing to release sluggish feelings so we may reveal the next layer. These soundings help us to become willing to take the action needed and desired.

Intentional use of aerobic sounds activates our internal *chi* so we can better tend to our own best interests. It is especially beneficial in moments when we feel stuck, tired, listless; don't want to take a walk, even though we know it's a great idea. Aerobic sounding breaks through our mental-emotional-physical resistance and awakens our own natural internal medicine.

The way that I begin most sounding sessions is to sound and teach others to release what is not theirs—to keep reducing ancient and current emotional residue stored in the tissue. We listen, respecting each layer, and we empty a layer at a time. We cultivate our willingness to express the unexpressed, that which may be running the show whether we have acknowledged its presence or not.

Emptying with sound is truly an invaluable tool. Sounding empties us of what is no longer needed or useful. We are releasing our own negative self-talk energy and that which we've gathered from others during conversations, television viewing, radio listening, or simply walking down the street. We are releasing a constant interchange of energies that "get stuck *on* and *in* us" daily. What is not mine and what is not needed, I let it all go, without analysis.

Analysis = Paralysis

Explore the languages of sound in your laboratory. How does your sounding affect you physically, emotionally, mentally? We only know how sounding works by making sounds.

Note: Additional Sound Vocabulary can be found in Appendix 1.

Chapter 4

Emptying

Whatever Is Unexpressed Runs the Show

Bodies taught me this truth decades ago: Whatever is unexpressed is controlling my actions and my thinking; "running the show" without my being conscious that this is occurring or is even a possibility.

Experience has shown me that if I do not have a personal means or a tool to express my impatience, intolerance, regrets, worries, or blames in a creative way, I become quite congested. I feel stuck and irritable, often ashamed of my situation and my inability to control this eruption of discomfort. My irritation will seep out in some way, usually at inappropriate times. My anger, regret, and jealousy come out in the most surprising ways, and often with people that it has nothing to do with. Then, of course, I feel embarrassed, apologetic, humiliated, or just rude, and this creates a need to defend myself, or cross the street if I see you coming.

These are mental gymnastics that can occur when we get too full, stuff things down too much, become scared and overwhelmed, without the foundation of an internal reserve. Every day, I practice sounding my whine as an emptying exercise so that I can show up as a woman of dignity. I do this emptying even if I do not know or feel like there is anything going on in my emotional/feeling body. I assume there is always hidden residual energy from my life interactions that can be emptied.

We sound to get QUIET,
to LISTEN to our Inner Teachings.
We empty daily to have more room
on all levels of perception,
physical, emotional/feeling, mental, and spiritual.
Sounding creates more internal room
to receive the sunlight of the Spirit,
to feel and to Be Light.

When Do We Need to Empty?

These are some symptoms of needing to empty—to let go of—that which is not our own:

- Never seem to have enough time
- Often agitated, impatient, irritable
- Don't know how I feel
- Can't rest deeply or enough; can't sleep
- Sensation of numbness, lack of presence, when we touch our body
- No one at home—got so crowded, we had to leave
- Processing or telling a story over and over
- Trying to "fix" what is not mine
- Energetic codependency; can't stay out of others' business
- I want to help; afraid they cannot help themselves without me
- After having an upset, an argument
- Being with many people, many conversations
- Emptying can allow the digestion of too many words in our heads.

There are many forms of emptying. Some people run, others walk, write, paint, dance, sing, drum, and sound. There are many creative forms that provide us the opportunity to empty. Find your own form and practice, often. It all works.

The Jaw–The First Emptying Gate

I have nothing but great respect for the power of our jaw. As humans, it was our first line of defense. The jaw is one of the strongest muscle systems in this body of ours. It nearly matches the uterus in strength. As above, so below.

The jaw tightens and takes on holding patterns for numerous reasons: being told to shut up or to not speak, being physically abused in any way, receiving a whiplash or head injury, having poor posture and misalignments of the spine, TMJ, surgeries, emotional pain and fears of any sort, the social restrictions and health fears experienced during the COVID-19 pandemic.

All of the above, and more, contribute to the jaw's tight holding patterns. It is trying to protect us from feeling our reaction to events, yet the events and the jaw tension are recorded in the entire body. This holding pattern in the jaw can inhibit the breath, restrict the spine, and lock the knees and ankles.

If we have had pain or surgeries, the jaw will try to help us get away from the pain, to lift up and away from the injury. Years later, the jaw may still be holding us back from pain that is no longer evident or present. In these instances, the jaw is behaving as a support system, holding us up as we move through the world. When the jaw is tense or held, it acts as a primary support system, like the feet.

For instance, without realizing it, our jaw may clench while we are carrying groceries, opening doors, driving our car, cutting vegetables, or writing a letter. You are invited to simply be aware. Our feet and pelvis are the weight-bearing parts of our body, not the jaw.

It is important that our jaw learns to relax. When we recognize tension in our body, it is wise to bring our awareness to the jaw. We can often relax and release whole-body tension from here.

I touch my jaw and cheeks, soothing them with *Shhhh, it's okay, sweetie. You can let go.* My hands give a cue that my jaw can soften. By the act of relaxing the jaw, our voice can rest deeper and be held by our breath, and the body can receive our sound and breath. This is most difficult when our jaw is set tightly. The holding creates confusion and conflict in the body and inhibits our ability to vocalize. I can't feel the rest of my body if my jaw is tight.

The first thing I want to notice for my own body, or the body of someone else, is if my jaw is held. If my jaw is held it inhibits my breath and holds me up out of my foundational support systems.

EXERCISE 1
Softening the Jaw with the Silent *AH*

This exercise begins the reeducation of how to relax and release holding patterns in our jaw. Please do not use effort.

- Gently open your mouth, and allow the *AHHH* to come out naturally, without any concern for pitch or range.
- Sound your *AHHH* in an easy speaking voice, even a soft whisper, to begin with.
- Let your *AHHH* shape and touch the roof of the mouth. Imagine the *AHHH* expanding your head's resonance chamber. Feel the sound vibrating in your throat.
- The roof of the mouth starts shaping and engaging the cranial structure and jaw.
- Feel the sound waves of the *AHHH* as it awakens the liquidness of your body.

EXERCISE 2
The *AH* Massage

AH is a most generous sound. Voicing it suggests that we open our mouth wide, allowing the *AH* to fill up this cavernous space, touching the roundness of the roof of our mouth and throat. The back of our head starts expanding and claiming its roundness, too. As we assist the jaw to soften, the entire body will receive release.

- Act as if your body is a liquid terrain and the shape of the AH vowel is shaping the inner terrain of your mouth.
- Let your breath help and support your shape of *AH*.
- Relax and notice how you are feeling.
- Repeat as often as you wish.

EXERCISE 3

Moving deeper into *AH*

The *AH* shape is a loving way to remember, to release, to relax, and after a while you may notice that your shaping of the *AH* is moving deeper into your body, down to your chest, including the space of your back, and maybe it starts shaping inside your abdomen. A most generous vowel, the *AH*.

This simple exercise will help you start retraining the jaw to relax and soften.

- Imagine that you are making the sound of *AH*.
- Let the shape of the *AH* be experienced.
- Do not make the sound out loud; simply imagine that you are making the sound.
- Feel how the sound of *AH* shapes your mouth.
- Notice how it starts rounding the roof of your mouth and softening your tongue.
- Let your breath help support your shape of *AH*.

The Hum as Integrator and Closing Sound

The Hum is used with aerobic sounds to integrate and assimilate work we have just finished. It is often used as closure for a section of work and provides space for the body system to pause and rest and reflect.

Consider using the Hum to assimilate a strong conversation or inner work you have been processing. Or, when you have given or received a beautiful healing session, bring in the Hum to integrate all that occurred.

*Humming soothes and lubricates all your sound work through
the layer that has been addressed and throughout the entire body.
The Hum is the integrator, assimilator, and soother of sound work.
It creates a coherency of everything you have touched.
The Hum completes a layer naturally.*

EXERCISE
Emptying

- Begin, as always, with the Hum.
- Whatever conversation is in your head, translate the words into sounds.
- Whatever emotions are present, let their rhythms become sounds with clapping, stepping, moving.
- Explore many ways of releasing.
- Do this release for approximately 20–30 seconds. No more is needed.
- Pause and notice your breathing. Notice what you are feeling and where.
- Then close with a Hum.
- Repeat these 20–30-second release soundings 2–3 times while alternating them with a Hum.
- Take time to sense what is taking place with your breath, and in your being.

Sound Increases Our Capacity for Breathing

Our evolutionary capacity is connected to becoming more conscious of the power of our breath with sound. We can't sound without breathing. We need very little breath to survive. Sounding makes it easier for us to breathe deeply.

Our focus with breath begins with the exhale. Let us exhale what we have inhaled. We may notice that we are often held in an inhale. One hears that the planet is in a state of inhale. Pandemics, crisis, traumas, accidents, illnesses, and so forth can create a condition of holding the breath. Even after the traumas are over, or are no longer an issue, our breath may stay in inhale without our knowing it.

If we exhale, the inhale then easily happens. Remembering that our body knows how to breathe, we then practice conscious breathing to educate and remind ourselves to release, let go, exhale.

We have to take time to practice reclaiming our breath on a daily basis. For my practice I like to lie down, getting out of the field of gravity. I exhale slowly following the inner terrain of my breath.

Our physical body is three-dimensional, an asymmetrical design and shape, with a spiral and curved terrain. We allow our breath to match our interior design. As with sounding we speak of "matching" the shape of the emotion, the shape of the wound, the direction of the entryway. In the breath we want to match the inner texture/tapestry of our body. We remove the linear, straight lines from our breath. Linear breathing creates a stress for our breath. We want to match our curved interior shape.

Exploring Sound and Breath Possibilities

Sound releases tension and stuck emotions within breath. I can use my *AH* sound and move within my chest cavity to massage and caress and relax my thoracic chest. I can direct my *AH* toward the direction of my front and expand to my sides and into my back. I can allow the *AH* to fill the space of my chest chamber.

I use my sound to awaken my lungs and thoracic cavity. I direct my hum into my lungs and chest area. The Hum can easily engage and interact with my thoracic and cervical spine, where the ribs insert into the spine and ribcage. The Hum and *AH* lubricate the spine and ribs.

I pause, take a few conscious breaths, and notice how I now experience my ribs, lungs, and my entire being.

Practice Reclaiming Our Exhale

Practice breathing exercises lying down. We allow gravity to assist us in resting and receiving. When we are reeducating ourselves or learning a new pattern, it is best to avoid navigating the gravitational field. We can surrender to gravity when we lie down to learn. In this surrendered position, we can more easily place our attention on what our breath is doing.

Remember:

- We do not force our breath. It is not about how big a breath we take or release.
- Our focus is on being conscious, listening, and following our interior terrain with our breath.
- Let us put a curve onto and into our exhale.
- Let our exhale go deeper inside and rest and glide on our inner terrain. No effort. We want to rest and follow our exhale as it glides and swirls and curves itself down toward the pubic bone.
- With our exhale, the ribs start moving down toward the pelvis and hug our lungs. The ribs rest onto our lungs.
- With our inhale our ribs open and expand.
- Let us allow our ribs to dynamically respond and cooperate with the movement of the lungs.

EXERCISE
Reclaiming Our Exhale

- Get out of the gravitational field; lie down wherever you are comfortable.
- Bring your attention to your breath. Notice what your breath is doing.
- Let your focus be on your exhale. Exhale what you have taken in.
- Let there be a little curve, a little jiggle, a little movement in your exhale. Let your exhale be easy.

- Focus on your ribs. Let your hands rest on your sternum. Feel the weight and sensation of your hands. Let your hands caress your heart.
- The weight of your hands reminds your ribs that they are opening and closing as you breathe. (*Oh yes, my ribs get to open and close.*)
- Use your hands to touch and guide and release tightness or tension in your ribs.
- Your breath will go anywhere you direct it; it is so cooperative. Act as if your breath can go there.
- Whatever surface your ribs touch, that becomes a teaching place. Your ribs get to open and close against the bed or floor or chair.
- Practice exhaling and inhaling against whatever surface you are touching.
- Feel the dynamic movement and fluidity of your ribs.

EXERCISE
The Evolutionary Possibility of the Exhale

- Get out of the gravitational field; lie down wherever you are comfortable.
- Bring your attention to your breath.
- Let your focus be on your exhale. Exhale what you have taken in. Consciously reclaim your connection to your breath.
- Let your hands rest on your upper heart and upper chest area.
- Imagine your exhale spiraling into the upper ribs. Take time feeling the small spiral of your breath moving into the upper ribs. Imagine a tiny seahorse on the waves of the breath.
- Let your ribs and heart just rest into your hands.
- Remember your lung lobes; breathe into your upper shoulders, front and back.
- Take time. Relax and go deeper into layers of release and connectedness.

- Your breath starts teaching you the evolutionary possibility of what is ready to unwind and connect.
- Be willing and grateful to participate with the inherent wisdom of your breath.

Sound Prayer

I give myself this day
to that which I know is greater than me,
greater than you, greater than all we together know and can see.

I give myself this day
to that which is greater than all my pain, all my sorrow.
I give myself this day
to that which is greater than all my joy, all my gifts.
I give myself this day
to that which is greater than all my gratitude, all my kindness.
I give myself this day
to that which is greater than all my fears, all my worries,
all that I am powerless over.

I give myself this day
to that which is greater than all that I have power over.
I give myself this day
to that which is greater than all that I love
and care about and feel protective of.
I give myself this day
to that which is greater than all that I hate,
disregard, or put off and away.
I give myself this day.
Thank you.

Sound as a Prayer

My prayers always begin by inviting Source to be within my heart, and that Source be between myself and another. I begin my day with emptying. I begin my day by allowing the sounds to come up out of my belly through my breath:

— as an *AHHHHHHHHHH*,
— as an *OHHHHHHHHH*,
— as an *EEEEEEEEEE*,
— as an UUUUUHHHHHHHH OUOUOUOU,
   OUOU AHAHAHEEE EEEEEE OHHHHHHHHH
   AHHHHHHHH,
— as a *HUMMMMMMMMMMM*.

The magic and beauty of the Hum as an ongoing prayer is that it soothes, clears, and massages our inner terrain. The Hum taught me many ways for its use. It reminds me of what I learned from my elders about plants and herbs. It is more important to learn 40 ways of using one plant than to know only one thing each about 40 different plants.

I let the Hum and other sounds pour out of me for as long as they need to. I breathe in, I breathe out. I relax and listen. Is there more chatter going on? Do I have more to empty this day? If so, I continue and include more vowels and consonants, increasing the variety of shapes and sounds. I give my Intention for this Sound Prayer to relieve myself of the burden of excess baggage, the committee chatter, and just "stuff."

I Have Nothing to Say

Or, I have too much to say.
Or, it really doesn't matter what I say.
Or, can I say what I say and be kind?
Yes, that is all that really matters . . .
Can I practice kindness?

Am I willing to practice kindness?
I do know I can more easily practice kindness
if I have taken the time to empty
whatever may be in the way of kindness.

Each day I must be willing to release that which is burdening me.
I often need to unburden me of me . . .
My "stuff" that I like and that I don't like . . .
I want "stuff," I need "stuff,"
what do they think (about me) "stuff" . . .
Unburden the "stuff" of self . . .
so that which is more of essential essence can be felt and experienced.
I have freedom to release the bondage of the "stuff of self."

Let me be willing to empty the noise.
Then I may drink in and receive the light
from within and the light from without.
A simple process like running ourselves through a sieve.
Straining the fluoride and chlorine and all the
many microbes and bacteria that water can get filled with,
that which keeps the water from being its essential self.
So, we refine it the same way, at least in principle, that I empty myself
of that which is not essential in my water-based system.
Daily, I refine my waters, filter my water of that which is not
of my essence.

Health Benefits of the Sounds of Laughter

Laughter is a de-stresser and the easiest form of meditation since it brings about relaxation in a pleasant way. Sounding and laughter instantly lower blood pressure in hypersensitive people; they stimulate the brain, expand and enrich the blood vessels with oxygen, and send more blood racing to the extremities.

Laughter and sounding vastly reduce the body's levels of stress hormones epinephrine and cortisol, which in turn relieves stress &

tension. Meanwhile, the happiness hormone oxytocin is enhanced, which triggers a spike in immune-boosting antibodies.

Laughter and sounding increase lung capacity and therefore promote the body's ability to store oxygen, the life force that helps us stay young and disease-free. This is good news for asthma and bronchitis patients. In addition, laughter raises the immunoglobulin antibodies in the respiratory passages, thus strengthening the immune system to protect the body from infections and allergies.

Twenty seconds of aerobic sounding in the form of heavy laughter can be considered a form of stationary jogging. It stimulates the heart and blood circulation, is equal to 3 minutes of hard rowing, and will burn up to 400 calories per hour!

Laughter and sounding increase endorphin levels in the body— endorphins are natural painkillers and greatly help in coping with the suffering from arthritis, migraine headaches, and muscular spasms.

Laughter is one of the best ways for us to "lighten up" and be released from fear's grip. Laughter and sounding instantly raises your energy by clearing away negativity, confusion, and mind chatter. Above all, laughter is the "shortest distance between two people" and improves interpersonal relationships.

Note: See References for information on Laughter Meditation with Laraaji.

The Whales

The whales came to me in Dreamtime over a period of a couple of months in 2003. I had suffered a terrible fall in Europe, and for nearly a year I was in deep pain and fear as I really couldn't walk for more than a few minutes.

I had received much work from masterful folks, and was doing all the inner meditative and contemplative work I had gleaned over the previous decades, and nothing seemed to be touching the core of concern.

One night in my dream, I was awakened deep within the ocean by whales surrounding me and vibrating their frequency into my body. They came to me regularly and were restoring me with frequency. I will always be grateful beyond words to these powerful beings, which took the time and energy to feed me, heal me. This is another reason I can easily sit comfortably and say I do not know, and I am grateful for the deep mystery, grateful for their teachings and their generous ways.

I was left with the knowing: Whales are our ancestors, and they can live without us humans. But can we live well without them?

A Call to Awaken the Stuck Arteries in the Heart

Let the sounds send air and oxygen
and wind and eagles into the heart waves,
let the waves hold them
and balance and bounce them to their navel,
let the sounds become liquid,
and let them sink to the depths of the dark,
deep waters where we abide,
so that we can join in this chorus of union.
Tell them how much we need their sounds—
Please sing your soulful songs.

Chapter 5

Honoring the Body's Innate Wisdom

"One can go as deep into this human form
as one can travel into the outer galaxies."
~ **Dr. Ida Rolf,** creator of Rolfing

When some of us began this work, during the Human Potential Movement in the late 1960s and early 1970s, we were immensely excited about the evolutionary possibilities of bodywork, the many awakenings and memories, and the therapeutic content that the body was ready and willing to communicate.

Masterful teachers, such as Drs. Ida Rolf, Valerie Hunt, Wilhelm Reich, Randolph Stone, Judith Aston, and Emilie Conrad, and many others who came before them and many others since, were suggesting, experiencing, and teaching the deep intelligence within our physical form. The premise from our experiences was that the physical form was a doorway to a variety of diverse perceptions.

The Evolutionary Possibility of Bodywork

When I look at a human form or a natural landscape, it presents itself to me as a composed piece of music, a piece of art, through color, shape, rhythms, textures, and of course, frequencies and multitudes of geometries.

Most spiritual teachings suggest that pain is the touchstone for all spiritual experience. In my own journey, my discomfort was informing me to examine my behavior, my thinking, my actions. My pain was a signal to become aware and begin looking within.

I must emphasize that our journey to wholeness is an evolutionary movement, not a static place of becoming fixed. Please do not make sound healing another "fix-it" tool! Let us remove the need to say this frequency is for this ailment and this sound for this body system. We have an opportunity to allow sound healing to remain a form of transformation, a possibility of evolution; to allow the fluid body to continue to change and rearrange our thinking, postures, and cellular memories.

Can I surrender to the power of not knowing?
I only do not know, because I know,
When you know, you know you do not know.
The more you know, the more you know you do not know.

I love sharing my excitement about exploring our inner galaxy. I invite your excitement about not knowing. I do not want to miss the opportunity of discovering what my emotional, physical, and spiritual bodies may be communicating, revealing a deep knowing in my tapestry, for me to explore, notice, learn from, and deepen within.

Let us note the beauty of our human fabric, of this body's beauty, as well as its possible teachings within its unfoldment. In sound work, I want to enter my body's world through a soft spot, an opening into this unknown fascinating place. I want to be curious and to listen and see what may unfold.

Our Fluid Body

"We are on a path of conscious evolution when we begin to understand that we are bodies of living consciousness, not bodies of matter. We are vibrational beings, and sound is a vibrational key for shifting our frequency and accessing different levels of consciousness."

~ **Deborah Van Dyke,** musical artist

Our physical body is a terrain of approximately 70 percent liquid. Our bony structure has a liquid element, and the connective tissue surrounding all our musculature, our organs, and our various bodily systems is fluid. Even our brain tissue is primarily fluid. As the body is affected by aging, disease, accidents or trauma, this fluid system congeals, congests, crystallizes, constricts, and becomes thick or more viscous.

I can feel when my body starts to hold stress and anxiety. When painful emotions and harsh physical impacts settle into my body, the shock creates a distress that impedes movement and circulation of all fluid systems. The stagnation arising in my liquid system creates an interior environment that attracts more congestion. In the process, I forget that all is liquid, or desires to be so.

In these situations, I pause and Hum.

As a bodyworker in the mid-1980s, I started seeing more circulatory stagnation in my clients and more nervous system concerns with the increase of computer use. This change in our biology happened so quickly.

Currently when all of us are "plugged in" electronically, we need to be more aware of maintaining our liquidity. Sounding the Hum silently or aloud can be very helpful as we sit at computers. Pause and move away from the screen, continue sounding. Pause to listen, use the Emptying exercise, and return to Hum again and again.

When there is a great deal of lactic acid in the fluid of the musculature, as the result of too much stress or too many electronics, circulation becomes impeded, and toxicity is easily created. As the body attempts to remove excess toxicity through the blood, it will often get stopped in the areas that have the lactic acid buildup (stress), injury, or general muscular pain. Our natural liquid system becomes blocked. All toxicity moving through the fluid can easily get lodged and stored at the place where injury and tensions are held.

"My research has shown me that when emotions are expressed—that is, when the biochemicals that are the substrate of emotions are flowing freely—all systems are united and made whole. When emotions are repressed, denied, or not allowed to be whatever they may be, our network pathways get blocked, stopping the flow of the vital feel-good, unifying chemicals that run our biology and our behavior."

~ **Dr. Candace Pert,** neuroscientist

All matter is frozen music. I invite us to imagine that this may be true—that we are frozen music, and as we listen, as we sound and vocalize this body composition, we become enlivened.

Let us invite all our senses to perceive our body as this resonating chamber. We listen and perceive from our cells, from our heart field, from our various nervous systems, from all our senses. We allow ourselves to view from soft visioning eyes closed or softly "not looking." We allow the body to reveal its shapes and colors and textures. We look from our inner vision. Let us "act as if" we can and do perceive from senses that we possibly cannot or need not articulate; rather, we allow ourselves to travel for a moment through this terrain.

We practice listening. We slow our breath, we pause, we listen—from our feet, from our heart, from our belly. We travel deeper into this terrain of the unseen and unspoken.

Let us not concern ourselves now with what we are seeing or perceiving; let us not break the connection by wanting to "figure it out." We want to visit and get to know this terrain, to become familiar with its nuances. We listen.

Do you hear that faint melody over to the left of the pancreas terrain? Do you feel or hear the beat of blood through the venous canal toward the right? Do you perceive the weeping, fog-like texture of pastels glowing and smoothly moving across that glistening arena and creating another canvas for yet another display of inner galaxies and worlds?

This is not the time—and may never be the time—for interpretations or questioning. This is the time for gratitude and, for a fleeting moment, enjoying the scent of honeysuckle arousing a summer feeling from long past. Yes, let us pause and breathe in this terrain. Allow a moment to regard our body as beautiful and miraculous, an infinite possibility of star plasma galaxies. Pause to be grateful that we are being allowed a view into our inner terrain.

One could say, and I do, that the human form
is a composed piece of music.

I recall reading about studies of microphones set up to transmit sound from the body and from art pieces in the 1930s and 1940s. There are many evolutionary pioneers in every form of human potential. Thank goodness for so many of the old Theosophists—Leadbeater, Alice Bailey, Madam Blavatsky, and Nikola Tesla, to name only a few.

These metaphysicians were telling us about color and shape; they were creating drawings of auric fields in various states of disease and health, emotional and spiritual energies, and depicting so many of our energetic bodies. So much exploration was being done and being known prior to World War II that has been forgotten.

> "The Om rightly sounded releases the Soul from the realm of glamor and enchantment. It is the sound of liberation, the great note of resurrection and the raising of humanity to the Secret Place of the Most High after all other words and sounds have failed.
>
> "Om sounded forth, with intentional thought behind it, acts as a disturber, a loosener of the coarse matter of the body of thought, of emotion, and of the physical body. When sounded forth with intense spiritual aspiration behind it, Om acts as an attractive medium, and gathers in particles of pure matter to fill the places of those earlier thrown out."
>
> ~ **Alice A. Bailey,** theosophical teacher

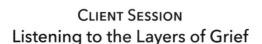

CLIENT SESSION
Listening to the Layers of Grief

A young woman client had many complications with her reproductive organs and eventually was advised that a full hysterectomy was the solution for any relief and future health. After her surgery, we began with the sound healing sessions.

- The first noticeable need from her body was to voice the rhythms of her overall physical pain.
- Inlaid and folded within was the grieving memory of the physical loss of her womb.
- And then many intricate layers of emotional loss of her body organs, the loss of the menses rhythm, and the grieving loss of childbearing.
- These are layers that are communicating simultaneously. The listening and sounding are going back and forth rapidly to catch the threads and integrity of the enfoldments of fascia tissue wanting to integrate and mend.
- Great anger and blame were present and revealed from years of incest.
- Psychological layers were twisted within her tissues regarding a belief that abuse caused reproductive cancers. Where and when would a layer of comfort arise?
- We paused and listened as her innate wisdom revealed the faintest hush of possibility and capacity for rest and acceptance, if only momentarily of a surrender to "what is" and the willingness to heal regardless of circumstances.
- This was the beginning of trusting a possibility for more and deeper healing.

Her story is a touching example of the innate, adaptive wisdom of our bodies. To heal and recreate ourselves over and over is always a momentous experience. The body wants to create life and healing through a spiritual solution.

Deep Listening

When we unwind holding patterns, traumas in the body, we listen for what is available first. We are listening for a doorway of entry, the soft spot.

Our listening and sounding is likened to the subtle opening of a safe. Turn a little to the right, then to the left, this sound, that sound—tones and pitches changing rapidly. We follow. The variety and diversity are immense. It is not symmetrical. Our healing and restoration follow the shape of our unique asymmetrical design or the design of the injury.

This is the reason we spend much time within our own laboratory, our own bodies, listening and sounding ourselves, our stories, our wounding, before we begin to listen to the complex math of unwinding the wounding of others. We learn to respect our own timing with acceptance and gratitude that our body is willing to communicate, and that we are willing and able to listen to its language.

Our work with sound is a constant formula of listening; observing, asking permission to be in communication with the rhythms, timings, shapes, colors, messages that our bodies wish to reveal. It becomes a sound print of textures.

EXERCISE
How to Listen to a Layer

- Always do a scan of the body before and after sounding. Walking, breathing, sensing pulses. Find some form of feedback for you and your client to help you recognize changes that arise from sounding.
- Always come with respect and acknowledge that we are touching an intelligent system.
- Ask or sense: Is there a place in this body wanting to express itself?
- Begin with Humming to create a cohesive canvas.
- Empty by sounding syllables, words, feelings, and unintelligible sounds.

- While sounding, notice when thoughts arise and return to the Hum.
- When you start thinking about anything (*When is lunch? What time is it? This is stupid. I like that sound. Maybe I'm a reincarnated opera singer*), or whatever thought floats through your consciousness, it is your cue to come back to your Hum and to digest that piece of work.
- I am sounding. I hear a thought. In this instant, I slowly start allowing the sounds I am making to find a curve, a turning point that spins and spirals me back into vowel sounds and Hum tones. I am bringing that layer home to be integrated. We are calling this "following and respecting a layer."
- Notice each time how you feel, what is happening physically and emotionally. If you feel there is more to tend at this juncture, you empty some more with the awareness. Go into a turning, spinning, spiraling path home to Hum and tones. Then pause and listen more deeply again.
- This is often done in three rounds. Usually, this is plenty for a session with self or another. Some sounding layers might be 10 seconds, some 30 seconds; rarely is it more than a minute.

Key Points for Sound as Bodywork

- We are listening and respecting the thin layers of fascia and the connections of one layer of fascia at a time.
- This form of listening starts revealing the accuracy possible for sound as bodywork.
- The ingredients of body layering formulas include rhythms, colors, words, shapes, timing, and frequency.
- The ancient teachings of respecting, listening, and following the pathways of wounding are the map to healing and mending one layer at a time.

One of the things I love most about this work is the continual wonder of it. I may think that I know what needs to be done, but when I start following the thread, the sound winds and travels and takes me to places

I never would have found if I'd gone directly where my mind thought it should go. I am always amazed at the power of sound, even after 50 years.

My Sounding Originates from the Blues

Blues that brought me to Surrender.
Surrender that brought me to Love.
Love that birthed the possibility to Live!
Before Love there were Blues.
Blues always brings you to Love.
If you follow the Thread.

Sound and the Physical/Emotional Body

As we seek wellness, we find that much of our pain, diseases, and suffering are related to emotions and experiences stored in our bodies. If you are a healing arts practitioner, you've likely had direct experience with this phenomenon.

Our bodies are intricate tapestries of weavings. This tapestry consists of fascia, tendons, muscles, nerve fibers, blood, cells, bone, all the ingredients and constituents that make up the physiology of our physical terrain, and it is repeated layer after layer.

If we sound the layer that is presenting, any holding within that layer begins to dissolve, to rest and regain elasticity. The next layer then arises and presents itself. By intentionally working one layer at a time, we help bring the body to a place of integration.

"I think unexpressed emotions are literally lodged in the body. The real true emotions that need to be expressed are in the body, trying to move up and be expressed and thereby integrated, made whole, and healed."

~ **Dr. Candace Pert**, neuroscientist

Chapter 6

Aligning and Tuning the Body

"If you change the alignment of a human form,
you will change the psychology of that person."

~ Dr. Ida Rolf

Science has demonstrated how sound changes the shape of water and
how sound frequencies create shapes and forms. Dr. Hans Jenny made
sound and vibration visible to us, through his Cymatics research and
recordings in the early 1930s. He gave us evidence that demonstrated
that frequency and vibration changed and rearranged form. Seeing is
believing.

*Even with all these facts and evidence that sound changes form,
this resonating principle can remain theoretical, separate from us
and from our bodies. We are a liquid system. If we sound,
we will change our form.*

Desiring to demystify this principle that sound can change and
rearrange form, I decided to use my own body as a teaching. I demonstrate how I use my voice "to tune" my body. This becomes a teaching
for participants with their own bodies as we continue our studies.
Seeing is believing.

Sound Changes the Physical Form

At the start of a sound healing training, I stand in the center of the group and give the students permission and direction to observe me. I ask them to notice how they perceive me now—my posture, my breath, my auric field. What has their attention? Then, for the students to notice how they feel as I walk by them—did they feel comfortable, afraid, anxious? Students gather some feedback for themselves before I begin tuning my body. They then see more easily what vocalizing does for the body.

This is a vulnerable position for me as a teacher. I do not know what will be revealed or what they will notice, nor do I know what sounds will flow through me and what within me is going to change and be rearranged.

I surrender to Sound as my Teacher. I remain curious and excited to experience how the sound frequency of my own voice sounding my body, can and does rearrange my liquid, my electromagnetic field, my "matter."

I begin with a Hum usually, in order to create an entering and a canvas. My body may direct me to a chakra center or identify a need to empty some congestion or undigested emotional feeling in my chest or abdomen.

I allow Sound as my Teacher to guide me, and I follow to the best of my ability. At times, my hands touch where my body wants sound. Often, my hands guide the direction or create boundaries for the sound. The body, mind, and sound are working as a unit. Sound travels around my body and my ethereal fields in numerous ways as I voice diverse formulas of sound. Unwinding and integration take place repeatedly. I am always amazed at the changes that occur. I never know how much I needed the tuning until I have tuned!

I have found that demonstrating is one of the more effective ways of teaching and making real the power of our voice, and people observing notice the changes that have occurred within me. It is most empowering to know that we each have this possibility within us to affect our physical, psychological, emotional, and spiritual self.

After sounding myself, I walk around the room in the same form as before the demonstration. Not only have students noticed changes in my physical and emotional posture but many also notice a change in their own breath and shape.

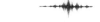

EXERCISE
Aligning and Tuning the Body

Scan the body before any sounding

- We always notice how we are physically, emotionally, psychologically, and spiritually before we begin our sounding/tuning practice.
- This is our laboratory, our body.
- Physically we notice as we walk about, how much weight do you feel at your feet?
- Is there more weight at the heel, toes, or to the sides?
- Is there a difference from your left and right foot?
- When sitting how much contact do you feel with the chair? How much weight do you feel in your buttocks?
- Is there a place in your body that wants your attention? Lower back, neck, knees?
- How are you feeling emotionally, psychologically? Sad, lonely, tired, anxious, confused, or contented?
- Spiritually, do I feel connected and calm?
- Am I breathing consciously?

Align and tune the body

- Begin sounding with a Hum to create an entering.
- Your body may direct you to a chakra center or identify a need to empty some congestion or undigested emotional feeling in your chest or abdomen.
- Where does your body need to sound?
- What needs to be expressed or assimilated? What does your body want to release or integrate today?

- Allow your hands to participate with the sound. Sound guides and directs you.
- Empty and Hum, empty and Hum.
- Close with your integrating Hum.

Observe the changes from sounding

- Pause and notice. Was there any change from what you observed before you started sounding? Take a walk again and become amazed at how sound works.
- Be specific, what changes do you observe in your body's laboratory?
- Was there any change at your feet, with your breath, your attitude?
- Does sound change your physical form and alignment?
- Does sound affect your emotional expression?

These are suggestions and keys for listening and sounding. I need to scan the body before I start sounding. This is the laboratory. I may jot down what I am aware of, so that I will recall after I sound and tune.

I have the upmost respect for Sound as our Teacher. I surrender to sound, knowing that it touches and works with our innate wisdom, and that the frequency, vibration, and resonance make the needed adjustments, if we allow, trust, and surrender to its teachings.

Tuning my body will enhance and expand the quality of my breathing, which increases oxygen and enlivens my tissue. Sound vibrates my bony structure, and in this dynamic process, it organizes and reorganizes my form to sustain a better alignment of my three-dimensional structures. I believe this is one of the reasons that sound is so effective for pain as it hydrates and oxygenates tissue.

Sound helps hydrate and lubricate all my systems. Sound vibrates my resonating body and allows me to move into a shape that is supportive in my core. It rearranges, expands, and reshapes where dimension and support have been diminished, ill-formed, and imbalanced.

As my body finds a better relationship to the present time, my emotional/feeling body is also changed and restructured along with the physical shape-shifting. Each time this occurs the experience is amazing, not only to the observing students but also to me. Sound is precise bodywork. Sound sets into motion whatever it touches:

- We know that our body is a resonating chamber and that it is 70 percent liquid.
- We know that frequency is a medium that activates the interplay or dance within our molecular structure.
- Science has articulated the process that occurs in the dynamic physical molecular structure.
- Physics shows us evidence that sound breaks up crystallization and coagulation.
- Sound changes and rearranges form.
- Scientists James Oschman, Candace Pert, and David Boehm describe energy vibrations, frequency medicine, and the vocabulary of how the rearrangement is an ongoing function of the life force.

Preparing for a Healing Session

Dear Body and Soul of Mine,
I invite you into my heart, into my life this day.
I want and need to have a relationship, a communication with you.
Please help me to know and to trust how to listen to you.
I pray to be your student. I pray to be teachable.
I pray to be willing to listen to your teachings of me to me, of you to me.

With a partner or client who has told you their concerns, begin with the following prayer:

I come to you my soul, my beloved.
I come with the concerns and inquiry for my friend (name).
I ask permission from the Soul, this body of (name).
What would you have me hear? What would you have me see?
What would you have me listen to?
I pray to be able to listen to what this body of (name)
wants us to know today.

Encodements of Forgotten Wisdom

Our *blueprint* is another word for our divine plan or the life purpose of our soul. Our *imprint* is what has happened to us in life. My constant prayer is that I follow my blueprint encodements and not get lost in my imprint.

This is the hardest part of listening to my soul's journey, because the imprint often seems more dramatic or enticing. Imprints hold trapped energies of past experiences, belief systems, wounding of a variety of sorts. Our ongoing work with sound is to sound the imprints that cover our connection in order to reveal our innate blueprint.

I experience with my mind's eye the ley lines within the body. I see the encodements as vortexes along these meridian lines. The vortexes have been a map of liquid light displaying the pathway of held wisdom. Encodements are wisdom containers that hold the memories of the past and the future: records of past lives, what we have experienced, and what is to be completed is revealed. They are a map of treasures. We listen for them. Our job is to unlock the holding mantles to reveal their teachings.

When I listen to the body, I am listening for the blueprints that are stored in the vessels of encodements. First, I sound or listen to the imprints of the superficial fascia that hold, protect, conceal, and reveal the placement of encodements.

Imprints are formed in our tissues from accidents; injuries of various kinds; our emotional, physical, psychological traumas; and our cultural habits. Sounding the imprints is needed as a daily practice. We keep sounding what the body wants to reveal, to dissolve the imprints that are covering up and protecting our blueprint encodements, our soul's purpose.

"The most secure place to hide a treasure of gold is in some desolate, unnoticed place. Why would anyone hide treasure in plain sight? And so, it is said, 'Joy is hidden beneath sorrow.'"

~ **Rumi,** Sufi mystic

Your Body as Your Teaching Laboratory

Your body is your teaching laboratory, your school. May that become increasingly exciting. Develop a daily practice of sounding, emptying, listening, praying, reflecting, and daily intention. Notice how your body, your life, is affected by your vibrational work. Use your voice to experiment and experience for yourself what happens within your physical and emotional state when you give voice to your body on a self-care basis.

The key to learning sound as medicine and bodywork is to know and understand how it works on you. If I do not know my own body and sound preferences, I cannot authentically be of help to others.

The more recent common approach to training practitioners is to focus on how to work with another person, but my experience tells me that if I know my own body and my own journey, I can more easily know yours. Also, I may cultivate compassion for how much energy, commitment, self-love, and time is devoted to creating change, to cultivating forgiveness of self and others, and to grieving those we love. It takes genuine willingness to walk this path of healing and awakening and not knowing.

Growing Heartful Possibilities

Most important in working with others is that we continue our own self-work. What a gift, what an opportunity. If you have decided to become a healer, it means that you have made an agreement to heal yourself. Ask yourself:

- Have I gone through my own healing crisis?
- Have I visited and embraced layers of my own shadow?
- Has my heart been broken by loss, grief, betrayal?
- Have I found compassion for my own human frailties?
- Have I gone deep into my well to find my Source?
- Do I trust, regardless of what comes my way, that I will be alright, whatever takes place?

- Have I forgiven as much as possible this day?
- Have I forgiven those whom I have felt betrayed me, abandoned me, and what I felt was not fair?
- Am I practicing a daily work of forgiveness and gratitude for the opportunity to be kind today?

May we all have loving kindness, tolerance, and patience toward all beings.

Listening to the Rhythms

What is the rhythm of the area you are touching or the area that is asking for your touch? Always begin with your own body. Become familiar with your rhythms, timings, and emotional shapes.

In classes, we sit around massage tables at a height that allows our arms to rest comfortably on the surface; the relaxed posture allows easy access for listening to our arm. We begin with listening to the rhythm of the ulnar bone and the tissue surrounding the elbow. We listen to whatever part of the arm calls to us, and then listen to the entire arm.

We practice trusting how and what the body wants to communicate, and we notice what language each of us perceives in. There is no right or wrong. We invite awareness. What are the rhythms each of us perceives?

I find that the more familiar you are with your own physical terrain, and the more time you spend listening in the ways described, the easier and more accurate is your trust in what you perceive in others. If you become well versed with your rhythms and preferences, identifying those of others becomes easier, too.

Keys for Listening to the Rhythms

This simple beginning provides an opportunity for listening and matching what we perceive. Notice how your body communicates rhythms.

- The first key of listening is love and respect.
- Practice acceptance for what you perceive without judging self or others.

- Our body may present rhythms of emotional memories, the rhythm of a knotted-up muscle, painful places, or rotated alignments.
- Bring attention to breathing patterns, where the breath is moving and where it is not moving.
- You may find your body sways or rocks to reveal the rhythms or movements.
- Perhaps you notice you are tapping out rhythms with your fingers or feet. The rhythm of an emotion or conversation. Become aware. Are your fingers or feet talking to you, demonstrating an unconscious understanding or communication?
- Trust your body is communicating on many different planes. Trust your body and learn how it communicates with you.
- Practice listening. How and what does the body want to communicate?
- Notice what languages of rhythm you perceive. Some folks perceive rhythm through color, shape, frequency, or sensation.
- Invite awareness. There is no right or wrong.
- How do you perceive the rhythms?

This practice becomes easier to relax into as we personally observe and experience the insights, inspiration, and transformations that are revealed when we surrender to that which we are—a human form learning to be in relationship and alignment with our Soul's purpose and grace.

EXERCISE
Listening to the Rhythms

- Start with a Hum.
- What is the rhythm of this day?
- What is the rhythm of your emotions today? Perhaps a staccato if you're in a real big hurry.
- Tap or walk the rhythms you perceive.
- Ask your belly, your heart, or another part: "What is my rhythm? What do I need today?"

- Become aware of how your body moves or wants to rock. Does your breathing change?
- Listen to your body. Notice: Are there areas that are slow? Areas that are fast?
- Ask your body: "What do you need here? Do you need me to slow down, or do you need me to speed up?"
- What feels comforting, soothing, pleasant, or easy for that part of the body?
- You are in a conversation with the rhythms of your body, your emotions, your thoughts. Pause and listen.
- Close with your integrating Hum.

The Physicality of Amnesia and Memory

Please tend to the desire and need to stay awake daily. Exercise the muscles and expand the nerve feed lines to activate and keep our fields of vision and wisdom shining in order to stay awake and be a beacon of memory.

The feed lines can easily become corroded. As mentioned, I started noticing this in my private practice in the 1980s with the increased use of electronics and computers. I was seeing this mucilaginous quality along the spine, especially as it seemed to originate at the cervical spine area. And it was covering the neuron-firing possibilities. I felt something was entering our bodies to "dumb us down," covering an impulse to awaken. I found that sounding work diluted this mucilaginous material and encouraged clients to do their formulas of sound therapy to keep their fluid systems more liquid.

These were my intense laboratory days in Chicago, where many practitioners were using many forms of color, frequency, breath, polarity, and radionics to work with themselves and others.

Sound nasally and in high tones toward the pineal gland,
then to the pituitary gland, and toward the brain stem.
Following deep inside the cranium is most helpful and
can keep a vibrational frequency for brain health.

Maybe I am mistaken, but it seems to me that by the mid-1990s those of us in the "alternative field" began to take a more conservative stance toward our work. Licensing issues and the fear of being arrested were commonplace, and some practitioners wanted to be recognized by the medical world and be able to take insurance. I understand this, but it seemed to diminish the pioneering possibilities of our work, except in small pockets of the US and beyond.

Yes, we were idealists, and may we continue to stay with the wisdom of this body and the nature she is created from. I trust that the younger folks will pick up on the immense possibilities of unification and evolutionary thinking.

The main benefit of vocalizing with intention and awareness is increased memory. I personally believe we have hardly touched the possibilities of voice and memory. The frequency of voice restores and maintains coherency within all our systems.

The first teaching Sound revealed to me, in the late 1960s, was that sounding helps us to remember. I started sounding as a young woman because it supported my need to wake up and stay awake—it was already obvious that it was easy to fall asleep or become numb or just get by, and that could happen to any one of us. I started sounding to stay alive and remain enlivened as if my life and the quality of my life depended upon it. I am grateful for the many folks that wanted to sound with me.

Staying Alive and Humane

How can I say, without alarming you, that we must pay attention to and cultivate our biological memory? How can I say, kindly but loudly, that all the hours, days, and years of eating laboratory-produced foods may have influenced our body chemistry and ability to remember our roots? How can I go into the impact of all the electronic modifications in our lives?

No wonder we have so much amnesia, so much greed. We have lost heart. How do we grow our hearts, especially if they have lost their memory? I trust that we can.

Sound, sound, sound! Sing your heart song, and keep a frequency and vibration tingling through your physical visceral being. In these times of living and our future times on this planet, it is more essential than ever for us to have a daily practice of self-care, self-awakening, and cultivating a willingness to stay awake.

May I Become Good Compost

"If you have any biology left in your body,
cultivate its life, grow some more biology."
~ **Emily Conrad,** founder of Continuum

Cultivating an approach to nutrition that feeds and nourishes our nature and body offers us the comfort of self-care. What is my constitution? What works for me? Am I eating food that my body can digest, that breaks down? Am I eating food that is compostable?

I am a licensed nutritional therapist. At one of the first residential trainings I offered, I bought groceries and created menus and pronounced to the class that it was necessary to learn how to cook and what to eat to become a sound healer! Blessed be, the students listened and took direction! I am not sure if that would be true today, that I could be so adamant.

There are no "seams" from one body system to another. Our whole being is influenced by the vibrations and energetics of the food we ingest. We assist our clients, not by saying you should only eat this or do this diet, but by addressing the basics. If your diet consists of sugar and coffee and few vegetables and digestible proteins, you possibly could experience anxiety, mood changes, depression, and pain. This is a broad statement, but often it is just that simple. You may need a nutritionist not a psychiatrist.

As long as 30 years ago, tests on human tissue were already finding it full of plastic and petroleum products. Morticians were noticing that they needed less formaldehyde to embalm bodies, as bodies were already self-embalming. Studies were showing that diet sodas were a major contributing factor. Consumers were led to believe that staying away from sugar was the way to live healthier, so artificial sweeteners became what was considered part of a healthy diet.

Decades ago, folk singer Woody Guthrie wrote the words, "Plastic doesn't reincarnate." This is a most serious statement.

If I have maintained a diet of additives, artificial sweeteners, artificial flavors, and artificial food that has never been in the earth or touched soil, I might find it difficult to feel connected to the earth, as I have become disconnected from my beginnings and my Source. Now, though, I want to become a sound healer, a massage therapist, or other bodyworker, because I know I have the ability and the desire and the love. So, I may need to listen with a different perspective to what kind of fuel I am giving this body of mine.

Dr. Liss, one of my first mentors, taught me about food and the need to eliminate life-depleting foods and lifestyles from my diet. He taught us to empty, eliminate, detoxify, surrender anything that was not life-giving in our food. As a healer, I need to hone my abilities to listen with all my senses, so I might need to get my pendulum out and check whether a particular food is right for me. (See Appendix for a biography of Dr. Liss.)

As much as possible, I am suggesting that you consume foods that have been alive, that have a life force, a rhythm, a pulse that feeds your dreams. What is the rhythm of your nutrition, the rhythm that influences your listening, sounding, and all your perceptions? Pay attention to your nutrition.

Chapter 7

The Heart and the Gut of the Matter

"In the last few decades, science has authenticated the presence of all living matter being housed in an electromagnetic field (EMF). Our entire world is one of polarities. Our planet, and all matter in one form or another, is held together and shaped by the attraction and relationship of an opposite current. Every cell of our body is surrounded both in and outside of its structure with electromagnetic energy. The relationship between this contraction and expansion, the interplay between this molecular dance and the tonifying result, creates our very form and shape."

~ Dr. Valerie Hunt, scientist

Our Energetic Roots in History

In the early 1900s, a young man named Nikola Tesla introduced the concept that the electromagnetic field surrounding Earth could be harnessed and used to fuel and give electrical power to our entire planet. He was suggesting that we would never have to dig into the earth for fuel to support the electrical needs of its inhabitants.

The industrialists of that era were not interested, as they could not afford to entertain possibilities such as those suggested by Tesla's work. It is said that when JP Morgan understood the magnitude of Tesla's vision, his response was, "If I let that boy have his way, I will end up as an antenna salesman!"

The very old disease of greed diminished our view of the power of nature and its wisdom. Our main task today is, and always has been, to stay awake and continue nurturing the memory within us of our connection and relationship with nature.

In the early 20th century, Western cultures began to slowly embrace teachings from ancient Asia focusing on the principle of electromagnetic energy flows (meridians) and polarities in the body. Starting in 1912, Randolph Stone, a doctor of osteopathy, chiropractic, and naturopathy, developed a form of bodywork called Polarity Therapy, influenced by both Eastern and Western healing traditions. He wrote about it for the first time in his book *Energy*, in 1947. Stone's work focused on pathways of electromagnetic correspondence throughout the body and the corresponding relationships of these points with the elements of nature. Shiatsu, jin shin jyutsu, and acupuncture are just a few of the other bodywork modalities that have provided a foundation for the electromagnetic healing approaches we often reference as Energy Medicine.

The Shaping of Our Listening

"The magnetic field produced by the heart extends around the body in a torus, a spherical shape that continually flows through space. The whole body is cradled within the electromagnetic field generated by the heart."

~ **Stephen Buhner,** herbalist and teacher

I believe that utilizing the heart field as a means of connecting, communicating, and sensing others is the medicine and means for healing overtaxed, stressed nervous systems. Utilizing our heart field for listening, perceiving, and connecting with others allows our autonomic nervous system to rest deeply within us. In our work, we practice not extending our autonomic nervous system in order to perceive.

I imagine that there will be a time when connecting through the heart field becomes our common form of connection. I trust we will mend generations of the physicality of codependent stress, rather than approach it solely as psychological codependence. The heart brain and heart field are the result of a complex unified expression called "brain coherence." Our bodies' receptors are designed to cooperate for the greater good.

People often ask, "How does one listen to the body?" and "How does one listen to what wants to be revealed?" We listen and perceive from our heart field. We allow our perceptions to touch what we are viewing. When we approach another from the heart field, our body perceives a spiral or curved geometry.

The heart is an organ of perception and communication, an electromagnetic field of love, to which all sentient beings respond. When we listen from our hearts, we receive and are received.

Listening from our heart field slows us down, and we enter the heart's space with respect. Listen for the soft place of entry. Respect for our spirally matrix creates a coherence of communication. Without words, the person feels heard, seen, and sincerely cared for energetically.

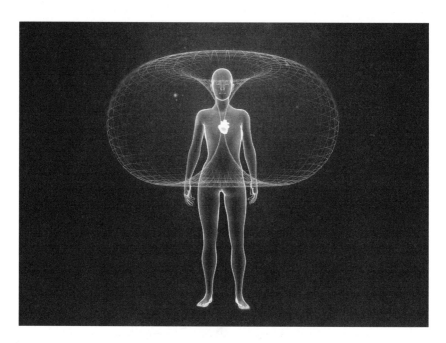

Toroidal heart field

A Curved Listening

The cochlea is our beautiful inner ear. We need to give ourselves a "curved listening," a shaping of a soft reception. As such, I want to cooperate with my shape. My listening needs to match the spiral shape and function of my inner ear. We are not linear.

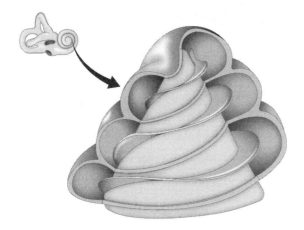

Cochlea

Notice the shape of the cochlea in the picture above. Our entire body field has a similar curved nature. Listening with all our senses and from our curved three-dimension, we want the body to feel heard. We are a three-dimensional body wanting to match, reflect, and resonate with another three-dimensional body.

How do you want to be met? A straight, head-on, linear approach toward someone often creates a holding of the breath, a reflex of moving away, a blocking from touch. These responses are nearly always involuntary and autonomic. I believe that communicating linearly can be interpreted as going against the grain, as if on some level our bodies do not feel received or heard.

Our intention is to reflect what we are touching. Let us soften the gesture of our hand as we approach another's field and allow a light arc of embrace. The body always responds in a more welcoming, opening manner when we enter its field with a slight curve.

Plugging into Earth, Ground Force Reaction

The earth we stand and sit upon is electromagnetic in nature. Simply, then, I wish to describe "plugging in" as a visual image of connecting with the electromagnetic field of the earth.

I acknowledge that all the nerve endings of my nervous system are easily accessed from the soles of my feet. As I stand or sit with the soles of my feet touching the ground or floor, I am plugging my nervous system into the nervous system of the planet. To sustain light, the lamp on your table needs to be plugged into the electrical circuits of your home (which are connected to the earth). In the same way, your body must be plugged into the earth to sustain its electrical vitality. From the feet up through the head, we experience a vertical grounding.

Most of us have ridden a bicycle or watched people riding. Call up this memory now. The sensation of our feet touching the earth is like pushing down on a bicycle pedal. Full footed, we go up a steep incline and as the pedal comes around, the field comes into us—right foot pushing, left foot releasing, and pushing again. Another example of this "felt sense" memory is the feeling of a cat kneading upon our chest or lap.

The earth is before me, beside me,
In front of me,
Behind me,
Above me, below me, inside me.
I can rest assured.

EXERCISE
Ground Force Reaction—Plugging In

You can always plug into that which supports your being and essence, no matter where you are—directly on the earth or on the floor of your 20th-floor apartment. Bring your attention to your feet and the ground/floor beneath them. If you cannot stand, bring your attention to your pelvis and sit bones. These are your base of support, the weight-bearing parts of the body. You stand on your feet, and you sit on your pelvis. Soften your jaw and remind yourself that you can be supported by the earth below you. You do not have to hold yourself up from the earth, the floor, or the chair. Let yourself rest into your support system. Use the examples of pushing on a bicycle pedal. We are an electromagnetic field and we live on an electromagnetic earth, so let us plug into it now.

- Rest onto the earth. Let the nerve endings at your feet "plug into" the electromagnetic field of the earth. Allow the tens of thousands of nerve endings at the soles of your feet to connect into this matrix.
- If seated, allow the nerve endings at the base of your spine to reach down and tether you to the earth. Feel the weight of your pelvis and buttocks resting on the chair. While sitting you can let your buttocks hug each other and release. This helps you to settle deeper onto the chair and pelvis.
- Use imagination to assist, if necessary ("act as if" you can be supported).
- "Plug in" as deep as the Grand Canyon and as high as the sun.
- Rest assured that you are held by the earth.
- Push down lightly and release upward as your feet touch the earth and the earth pushes back, imagine how a cat kneads.
- Rest into the support that you are standing or sitting upon. Your whole body relaxes.
- Practice daily letting the earth support you.

My focus with sounding, speaking, and singing is to have the earth support my voice. Grounding into the feet we invite the nerve fibers in the whole body to relax. The deeper I ground, the more I lengthen and increase my verticality.

Grounding, or plugging in, is not a static movement. We are grounding into and onto a planet that is alive and moving. We are practicing riding this wave. This same electromagnetic field can energetically be plugged into from our hands, head, heart, feet, or any part of our body. There are several energetic directions and geometries for connection and support.

Feet Brain

Standing on the bones
and listening to
their music.
Sitting and standing where you are . . .
Listen to the bones of life under your feet.
Listen to the rocks, the minerals,
all that we stand upon.

Your feet have taken in the pulses, the stored memories,
the information from everywhere you have walked upon this earth.

The "feet brain"—the nervous system at your feet,
All the nerve endings of our body are held at our feet.
The wisdom of the earth is at our feet.
We listen to the rhythms that we perceive from our feet.
We tap it, we respond, we invite,
we let it ignite us, we fill up with light.
The bones glow when they get noticed.
They turn into glowing heat of firelight signaling us on,
energizing us
to trust the earth.

Grounding and Stabilizing Our Circuitry

"The heart is an electromagnetic generator, producing a wide range of electromagnetic frequencies; an endocrine gland, making and releasing numerous hormones; and a part of the central nervous system. It is, in fact, a brain in its own right."

~ **Stephen Buhner,** herbalist and teacher

"Grounding" is a word that is often used in terms of electricity. We make sure we have a grounding rod to protect our appliances, computers, and all electrical needs. Damage can arise if there is no grounding rod. We can blow fuses, overload the circuitry, burn out cable connections, or start fires.

When we apply this concept of grounding rod to our own field, we protect our own state of health and nervous system; both are dependent on and influenced by our capacity to be plugged into this planetary matrix. Our wiring becomes tangled up, twisted, or even disconnected as the result of anxiety, depression, accidents—life experiences that impact us emotionally or physically. These experiences rearrange our structural alignment and often disconnect our energy.

The nerve endings at our feet plug into and receive signals from the earth. The "feet brain" then distribute these sacred vibrations upward through the body. Our intention is to have the earth support our voices, our sound vibrations.

The more the earth supports our body, the more freedom and ease is available for our breath, lungs, chest, heart, and voice. There need never be any stress in our throat when vocalizing. We are supported by the earth. Let our feet be present under our sound.

"Plugging in" reconnects us when we have become disconnected. Our connection to the earth rebalances our fields, our nervous system, and stabilizes our circuitry. This efficiently brings us toward coherence and balance. The more we practice this connection, the more likely we are to stay engaged and to continue mending and tending our communication with the nature that we are.

We often perceive grounding as a fixed unmoving position.
I am suggesting that we intentionally practice grounding as
a dynamic action. Our alive dynamic form is being
plugged into an alive dynamic earth.

EXERCISE
Ground Force Reaction and the Heart Field

Ground Force Reaction (GFR) helps us get into our heart field. The more we plug in, the more dimensions we can perceive. Our voice and Hum are also supported, our resonance changes. Humming into the heart helps expand the heart field. Imagine the electromagnetic field around our beings. The Hum increases our magnetic abilities. The Hum can activate and expand the dimensions in the pathways we have been exploring.

- Use your feet to "plug into" the earth below you.
- Feel the Ground Force Reaction coming into you from your feet and the earth below.
- Sound your Hum, and feel it generate and stimulate the tissues inside you.
- Visualize your Hum perceiving, allowing, being moved, and rearranged by the vibration of the sound currents.
- Your Hum sets up an action of movement, of fluidity. Feel the waveforms throughout your body.
- Using your hands, move this "felt sense" throughout your body.
- Notice how effortlessly sound vibration travels through your internal nervous system pathways.
- Imagine and sense the frequency throughout your entire nervous system and out through your spine, head, hands, and feet into the earth.
- Feel the frequency encircling and touching the membranes of the expansive field that is you.
- Sense the frequency of your Hum vibration touching, activating, and strengthening the perceptions of your heart field.
- Trust that by being connected within your own dynamic circuitry you can rest onto and into your own field of light and sound.
- Notice if there are ways you feel more present or secure.

Let Your Feet Brain Talk to Your Heart Brain

When I practice perceiving from my electromagnetic field, I can perceive and observe more clearly the pathways of currents moving throughout my body. The pathways of frequency are more easily sustained for vocalization. The electromagnetic field sustains me.

Let your feet brain talk to your heart brain. When we engage our heart brain, it invites communication with our gut brain and our upper head brain. We expand our capabilities to perceive and receive the information from the matrix of the earth's electromagnetic field.

Journey into the Inner Terrain

My experience of listening from the heart field reveals pathways of passages for light and sound to move through the body. These inner pathways light up. A map is revealed. These sympathetic and parasympathetic nerve pathways allow communication and information to flow freely.

The more I utilize Ground Force Reaction, the more easily the pathways are revealed. When I travel within these interior terrains and plug into the fields of support, I can sustain the three-dimensional volume of passages, and it increases the light quality—like pushing a button on a lamp or flashlight, to increase the span of light, or volume of light, or geometry of light.

The more plugged in I stay, the more present I am. It keeps me grounded and protects me from floating away and becoming distracted by the lights and colors and beauty that prevail within these inner world terrains. I observe the inner passages and my intention is to be tethered to this earth as I travel within these inner galaxies.

I want to stay conscious as I am altered within this perception. Within this altering terrain of circuitry, I listen and observe from my heart brain, and more "light" is revealed and made available. I imagine and visualize this taking place until I can truly perceive, in three-dimensional volume, those pathways that have always been there.

Imagination is one of our more powerful medicines. These visualizations and exercises I trust will birth and awaken new terrains of possibilities. This self-realization releases the world of theory and becomes a direct knowing—the knowledge of the nature we are. Our desire is to become students of our inherent and our interior nature.

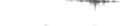

CLIENT SESSION
The Language of the Heart

In the late 1980s, I started working as a sound therapist at Dr. Ed Wilson's pain clinic in Boulder, Colorado. His clinic and research lab housed a chiropractor, a Rolfer, a Jungian analyst, a massage therapist, and me, an Aston Patterning teacher and sound therapist. We were all working cooperatively with a variety of diverse modalities for the good of the patients in various circumstances. What a wonderful, learning experience Dr. Wilson provided.

Dr. Wilson's patients had debilitating, life-changing pain resulting from accidents, surgeries, and various traumas that had altered the quality of their living. Pain had incapacitated their functioning life. He was a devoted researcher and wanted to know what were the results of using sound frequency medicine for his patients.

His laboratory was equipped to measure and record frequency changes, heat, emotional shifts, blood pressure, and the pulses of patients. Several times, Dr. Wilson would hook his patients up with electrodes and have me sound while he observed what was occurring in his instrumentation. This was reaffirming for his research and confidence-building for me. Concrete documentation was produced that sound frequency could change the pain receptors, soothe inflammation, and change perception.

One research patient gave me an immense teaching on the power of listening. Dr. Wilson had a laboratory, separate from our working clinic. He wanted me to work with a specific client. He asked me to stay outside (not even in the building) as he prepared our client by hooking him up to electrodes, blindfolding him, and putting him in a comfortable position.

Dr. Wilson then called me into his adjacent office and said, "Okay, here's what I want you to do: I want you to open his heart center!"

I just laughed. I said, "Ed, you are a totally radical, outrageous Scientist Being, but you often think in terms of your medical training. I do not 'open heart centers,' Ed. I do not know what his heart needs, and I would want to notice how his heart center is being supported and how his heart center is being secured."

Dr. Wilson looked at me as if I was speaking a foreign language and said, "I don't care what you do. Just open his heart center!" We had a deep trust and respect in one another's abilities, even though we had arrived from very different backgrounds.

He took me into the laboratory. The young man was lying down as I described above, with electrodes at his wrists and temple areas, and his eyes were covered. I start sounding his body, listening to what his form was displaying to be expressed. After a few minutes, the young man started crying and touching and patting his heart, crying and *ahhhhing* and speaking a language I did not understand.

Aha! Dr. Wilson and his technicians were all joyous as they exclaimed, "You opened his heart!" The mask comes off. The young man looks at me, holds my hand and says in English, "You were singing in my language." I believe it was a Czechoslovakian dialect. He was a student at Colorado University and had been away from home and his language for several years. The rhythms of the sounding matched a familiar cadence of language that resonated with him. This often occurs for the person receiving sound.

Now the scientist inside me says, *Ummmm, if I am away from my native language, the language I heard when I was in the womb, and it has been years since I have heard this language, when I hear it, it touches me, it touches my heart.*

The teaching of this session that touched me so deeply was the power and accuracy of listening that comes from plugging into the earth and matching the rhythm that this man's body wanted to reveal, and I believe what this man's heart was needing to hear. When we follow the listening, the rhythm, as best we can, the body will reveal the formulas and formations needed to receive its healing frequencies.

When we listen to what desires to be expressed, we touch the inner needs and the well of wisdom of the person we are sounding.

Surrender to Not Knowing

We do not need to know what needs to be expressed. We surrender to not knowing and trust with each person that if we sincerely desire to listen and communicate, to be in relationship with this soul, we will express what is being revealed. We do not enter a session with an agenda to "open" the heart center. We need not embellish, enhance, protect, or judge, what is being expressed. Our focus with sounding is matching a resonance that wishes to be expressed. It is gold for the person being received. If we sound authentically, the heart will open on its own.

Reminder of Essential Tools for Listening

- Love what is.
- Respect what is.
- Appreciate and accept what is.
- Ask permission to enter and listen, every time.
- Let the body know your intention to touch, sound, listen.

- Have the desire to be in relationship with what is.
- "Act as if" it is completely natural, reasonable, and possible to have a listening relationship with our self and others.
- Plugging in, grounding.

What I've Always Wanted to Say

Che ka ma so la to me la so ke la Che ka ma so me la—
mot el la Che ka ma so ka la
—mo te la Che ka ma so ka la—mo tel la

I've always wanted to say . . .
the language of the DNA is written in the fabric of the tissue,
inside the muscle, within the visceral sensation of the cellular threads.
And, it is a mending melody of remembrances and connections,
connecting our fibers with one another continuously.
The frequency of our being communicates with all other beings
through the thread of biological intelligence.

I've always wanted to say . . .
Do you hear the rhythm of your Soul communicating with mine?
Could we please get underneath our language and listen?
to the intelligence that rarely gets to speak—
That rarely is sought.
We keep giving more words to describe that
which words cannot describe.

I want to say listen—
Put your ear to your belly, to your heart, to your spine, to your feet
and act as if you are alive and there is movement
communicating within your very essence.
Communicate your very essence
that is relating to me, that is relating to you
I touch you, you touch God,
God touches me, I touch . . .

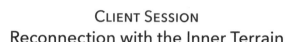

Client Session
Reconnection with the Inner Terrain

"One becomes aware of an inner electrical equilibrium."

~ **William Tiller,** scientist

One day I was doing some deep inner exploration, working within my own body, tuning, emptying, and listening, when I heard this strong crying in my womb, my abdomen area. I sensed a young child. My first action was to ground into the earth (plug in), listen and inquire, look inward. I needed to let go of any "story" or fear my mind wanted to go into. I needed to trust and seek solutions.

I felt much fear from her, and then I started "sensing" all around her and found her to be disconnected from the whole fabric of her physical being. She was living fragmented. She was unhooked from any stability. She had the sense of being abandoned as she wasn't plugged in!

With visualization and imagery, I started "plugging her in"—into the tissue, the terrain of her womb, into the abdomen in which she was residing. Connecting her from her back, sides, front, head, and toes. The more she became connected, the quieter and more comforted she felt. And then I watched as my body's membranes started covering her and enclosing her into the fabric of my being, her nature. She would no longer be fragmented from the whole. It was as if she was being wrapped in a baby's receiving blanket.

I have no idea how long she may have been in this state of disconnect before I was aware of her presence or how much had to be dissolved before I could perceive her distress. I had to do a lot of emptying and inner work with sound before her distress was even revealed. This is how

122

a section of fragmentation is revealed during a session. Sound dissolves that which covers and protects what wants to be revealed and healed.

Babies feel very insecure and abandoned when they are left with arms flailing in the wind. We need and want something to push against, to feel our boundaries, and get our footing.

I was utilizing my heart field to perceive her inner self, which was in distress. The heart field gives perspective and objectivity for perceiving inner and outer terrains. One has opportunity to see "holistic medicine" in action. Not only does one treat the physical body when working with this system but the psychological and spiritual realms as well.

We witness the interaction between body, mind, and spirit in healing. We utilize our imagination to travel where we may not know, by "plugging into" the support of the nature that we are.

The Mysterious Nervous System

In *The Science & Art of Herbalism*, Rosemary Gladstar wrote the following:

"The nervous system is the primary interface between the physical body and the greater consciousness of the Universe. If that is all there is to the nervous system, it is enough to make it, far and away, the most important system of our body. It is what provides integration and coordination to our lives. It allows us to see, feel, touch, act and react, create. Without this basic physical nervous system, there could be no life. To the degree that it is impaired, the quality, tone, color, and richness of life are diminished. If for no other reasons than these, we must commit ourselves to keeping our nervous system healthy if we want a full life . . . If we are suffering pain or distress to the nervous system, it is a warning of imbalance or danger to us. Pain is simply a message that there is something I need to be listening to physically, emotionally, or mentally."

Parasympathetic Rhythms of Breath and Sound

One of the main attributes of the parasympathetic branch of the autonomic nervous system is that it allows repair to take place within the entire nervous system, which can mend, restructure, and relax itself. The parasympathetic is engaged during our reflective and meditative practice. This is one of the truly important life-giving actions of the art and science of meditation: it trains our nervous system to be in the parasympathetic state. It enables a state of restfulness, rejuvenation, and repair, and provides the ability to listen and assimilate physical, emotional, and mental processes.

Just as the parasympathetic gets you ready to *BE*, the sympathetic nervous system gets you ready to *DO*. The sympathetic turns on active functions—physical activity and movement, mental planning and creating. These intelligent systems work together to support all our life experiences.

The parasympathetic nervous system is what allows us to digest our food and assimilate nutrients. Many of us have the memory of when dinnertime became the terrain of arguing or critiquing in some way. Others spend time dining while watching the news on TV. It has become the norm to "eat on the run," driving and multitasking while eating. I am sure each of us can identify some of these habits in ourselves. These habits send our nervous system into stress, into overload.

Digestive issues often start at a very early age and form a stressed pattern in the nervous system. A stressed digestive system creates a myriad of lifelong digestive conditions. We know the importance of our parasympathetic system in overall health, in being able to digest food, as well as digest multitudes of information that come into us daily.

Activating the parasympathetic system helps mend and repair the digestive system. Parasympathetic resonance reeducates our nervous system. The parasympathetic breath and sound exercise does the reeducating naturally and easily.

EXERCISE
The Parasympathetic Breath and Sound

The following exercise will aid in reeducating the nervous system. Supporting the stressed nervous system to slow down enough to be entrained to the parasympathetic rhythms and patterns.

Note: My gratitude goes to Emilie Conrad for her influence in this exercise.

For several years, I wanted to have the experience of sound and breath having more "felt sense" inside of my body, more sense of weight and inner touch. I wanted to more deeply experience the texture of sound touching my organs and skeleton inside me. This exploration guided me to the deep relaxation of touching the parasympathetic system.

Our intention becomes the "felt sense" of weight within our body, or more specifically along the frontal part of our spine. The imagery is to touch our spine area with our breath and sound. The focus will be in and around the front part of the spine. Beginning at our throat and touching the pathways of the dorsal vagal nerve and spiraling slowly with our hand down the front of our spine to our pubic bone. Our focus is to touch inside our body more consciously with our breath and sound.

We envision impressing upon and within our interior landscape, touching the landscape with resonance and breath. Our intention is to let the body receive and sense being touched, molded, shaped, and massaged by our breath and sound—truly touching the inner edges and inner shapes.

Please remember that we give our bodies our intention. Our bodies know exactly where the vagus nerve is, where the nerve endings are in relationship to our spine. We need not know with our mind. Please trust that our bodies know.

The Parasympathetic Breath and Sound exercise has six rounds:

- Sit comfortably with your back comfortable on a chair or cushion.
- Your focus and intention are going to be upon the front part of the spine, on the parasympathetic nervous system. **This is done very slowly.** Rounds 1-3 are done with an audible exhale.
- Begin at your neck/throat area, your hands touching lightly at the base of your ears. Slowly and gently move your hands to your throat.
- Make a spiral circular movement with your hands.
- Your breath is an audible exhale, like a whispered *"ah."*
- Your hands synchronize with your exhaling breath in a spiraling way.
- Beginning at your throat, slowly move down the front of your body, following the path of the inner spine.
- Your hand moves as it follows your exhale. When your exhale is complete, pause where you are, then inhale. Continue along the front of the spine on the next exhale.
- No hurry. This can take many exhales to find your way down the front of the inner spine.
- When you reach your pubic bone, pause. Take another inhale and exhale, take time to notice what may be occurring within you.

Round one is complete.

- Repeat this breath exercise two more times for the completion of three rounds of breath.
- In between each round, pause and breathe. Notice what is occurring.

- During rounds 4-6, add an effortless sound.
- Envision the *Ah* resting at the back of your throat.
- As you sound, envision touching and audibly massaging the front of your spine. Audibly massaging—*Ahhhing*—travel down the spine, vertebra by vertebra, from throat to pubic bone area.

- Remember the sound is one that is effortless for you.
- Pause, breathe, and notice how that feels to you.

Round four is complete.

- Use the same intention and focus for two more rounds, from throat to pubic bone area.
- The focus: Sound, as with breath, has a resting weight that deeply touches your interior. This is done slowly.
- With practice, you travel deeper into the terrain of your body.

After the six rounds are complete:

- Sit quietly and return to an easy, natural breath.
- This can be a gentle, helpful bridge into meditation and relaxation.

The result of practicing parasympathetic breath and sound: Being able to trust what you are sensing and perceiving. You can rest now. Rest assured that you are held and loved. Rest assured that you are supported by this earth. Trust you are held and loved by something greater than yourself. Rest assured.

Note: See Appendix 3 for information on my downloadable album *Rest Assured: Parasympathetic Resonance.* The album invites intention to rest, to entrain, to restore, and to remember how to live within the para-sympathetic nervous system.

Let Your Gut Brain Talk to Your Head Brain

"The Enteric Nervous System is another important brain that is immensely part of this complex unified expression called brain coher-ency. And it may be connected to that which we have called 'intuition' or 'my gut feeling.'"

~Michael Gershon, M.D.

Our second brain is in the gut, the enteric nervous system. Inner conflicts often come from not listening to the gut. My gut brain and head brain want to be in communication. If I don't have a relationship between my gut and my head, I am split. I need to have more cooperation between my upper brain and lower brain. How do they cooperate and listen to each other?

I am wanting to build a relationship between my feeling, emotional body, "my gut sense," and my more rational mind. These systems complement each other. I am wanting cooperation with my upper brain, my lower brain, and all the intelligent systems in my body. These are not higher and lower in terms of consciousness, just in terms of position in the body.

Often the head brain is not used to being in relationship with the gut brain. The gut brain rebels after a while. When my nervous system in my gut gets locked up, that affects the whole body. Digestive issues are epidemic because we don't understand how the nervous system and the gut fit together.

Wake up the communication channels! Sound moves throughout the entire nervous system. Every part of us is communicating with and coordinating with all the aspects of our digestion. When my head brain and my gut brain are in sync and have been listened to, my nervous system relaxes.

Exercise
Let Your Gut Brain Talk to Your Head Brain

Be kind to yourself. We were mental for so long. Let us give attention to the intelligence of the body. Start gathering that there is a brain in your gut—the enteric nervous system. Get that simple as a place to start.

- Speak your desire to have your gut brain and your head brain be in dialog with one another.

- Get a sound going back and forth between the gut brain and the head brain. Wake up the communication channels; giving it expression, giving it a listening. Allow the exchange—above to below, and below to above.
- Greet the different characters. Your gut says this, then your head says that. Notice who is talking first, who is needing what.
- What do you want to say, belly?
- Let your head brain tell your gut brain what it is up to and what we need to do.
- Let your head brain vocalize and verbalize your lists and instructions, or write down the lists so you don't have to hold it inside any longer. The gut brain loves to know what's happening, and it can relax!
- What does it sound and feel like when your head brain and gut brain feel listened to?

CLIENT SESSION
Myself, Shingles, and the Power of the Silent Hum

Shingles is a common, very painful burnout of the nervous system, caused from a stressed-out system that shows up as blisters on the body. Upon returning home from a two-month journey of traveling and working in Ecuador and Argentina, I awoke to find that I had shingles.

I had treated many friends and clients throughout the years, but I had no idea of what it was to have my nervous system so compromised by shingles. It is very difficult to be comfortable. Clothing, bedding—all are painful to the touch. Of course, this varies according to where one has shingles. Mine were on my right upper body, arm, and neck. I knew I needed high dosages of lysine and clay and cabbage. Cabbage poultice helps cool the burning sensation and restore a more alkaline environment, as does soaking in oatmeal baths.

My nervous system has always been a teacher for me. I was probably born with a compromised or had an already stressed nervous system by an early age. Having the ability to perceive energetic qualities without having any boundaries or discernment weakened and stressed my system. The nervous system registers "too much sensation; I am on overload." I have noted this as a common symptom to one degree or another in everyone with a highly sensitive system, those in traumatized environments, and a multiple of other reasons.

One of the symptoms of shingles I experienced was the stress of listening to words. Listening to conversations, television, telephones, even reading could be too many words; the words would activate a "doing" in my system, when all it wanted was to rest, not figure out words. Words taxed my stressed sympathetic system. Loud noises, machinery, lawn mowers, leaf blowers, and the like seemed to keep my nervous system agitated.

Some people sail through shingles, seemingly without being in much pain or having the sensitivity I am describing. Some of us have more challenged systems, and I am one of them. What was the teaching that my nervous system was giving me? It needed to rest. It stopped me.

During this time, my meditation, reflection, and mantra practice would ease my mind and quiet the injuriousness of the nervous system. After some time, I started sensing a drone-like sound coming from my deeper layers, an internalized Hum trying to engage me consciously. My inherent body wisdom was Humming, was mending my inflamed fibers.

What I was sensing was my Silent Hum, droning and getting my attention to help me. I believe this was revealed and accessible as the result of many years of sounding, working with myself and with my voice. My body had the memory and resonance of what was needed. I know this is how our inherent wisdom works, and it's a beautiful example of why we should practice. Repetition is so important. Even when I could not consciously remember, my body did, and came through the frozen fear to remind me of my healing abilities.

My healing ingredient was the Silent Hum. I have always held the power of the Silent Hum in the highest regard, but now it entered a level of "starhood" as it demonstrated the finest ability to weave, mend, nurture, and lubricate the fabric of the nervous system.

The formula of its rhythmic weaving was precise. I only had to completely surrender to its frequency and not attempt to direct or instruct. I simply needed to allow the resonance of the Silent Hum to mend and weave the fascia fabric of my nervous system. Sound is the teacher.

Speaking months later with a colleague who was just getting over the blisters from shingles and was still quite exhausted, I suggested she do the Silent Hum. She asked what that was. I told her that it's like humming a tune in your head—just include your entire body. Immediately, she experienced how soothing it was. It works. The Silent Hum is a compassionate nurturer.

Practiced regularly, the Hum increases its magnitude and creates a stronger magnetic field, as I experienced in my time of need during my quiet meditation time. Our magnetism of self grows, and it becomes easier to bring ourselves back home. The resonance of our magnetic energy draws our nervous system back into our body. I never underestimate the power of the Hum.

I experience silent sounding as more powerful and accurate than the audible sound. This accuracy is the result of much inner work practice in my own body laboratory.

Silently sounding trains the mental body to focus and listen to a wider band of frequency. The silent sounding can reach places in my body and follow interior nuances within my tissue and geometry. It becomes easier to recognize the direction of release and unraveling of holding patterns. The silent frequency can listen into crevices and corners of holding. It can easily follow a layer and change frequency effortlessly. Silent sounding can create tones and frequencies my audible voice cannot match, silently I can employ three to five frequencies at once!

I have the utmost respect for inner silent imaging possibilities. This could be very helpful in touching into blood vessels, tubular vestibules, sinus passages, and neurological pathways. I can become an explorer under water and find hidden treasures, claiming and reclaiming my interior dimensions.

Chapter 8

Dissonance and Shadow Work

"In the sounds of Asia, Japan, China, and India one can hear the power of the contrasting timbre of seemingly untuned instruments. These resonances have holistic quality based not on mathematical tuning but on the quality of the psychic feeling-response they are meant to elicit. The sound bipolarity of Tibetan cymbals, Balinese gamelan, African gongs, Amerindian drums, and Peruvian whistles, to mention a few, are often heard in shamanic rituals, and they lend themselves to the expression of emotional bipolarity such as calm and anger, love and hate, harmony and disharmony."

~ **Dr. Elide Solomont,** composer and psychoanalyst

Due to the unfamiliarity of the sound, Dr. Solomont suggests that dissonance can evoke unfamiliar and disowned parts of us, the shadow, where the ego is not directing. It is only in accepting and working through the shadow that we reap long-lasting results, in which we feel integrated and whole.

"The unfamiliar sounds of dissonance may evoke one's unfamiliarity by transcending known feelings and memories and excluding personal issues and problems. One may accept the dissonance or reject it. If accepted, one's ego may surrender to the experience, thereby transporting us to altered states. Dissonance becomes an object of contemplation. We turn inward, we let go and surrender. Cultures throughout time have used drugs, dances, and music in their ritualistic ceremonies and problems were solved in a non-linear manner, and spirituality, as self-actualization was experienced."

~ **R. Radocy & D. Boyle,** *The Foundations of Musical Behavior* (1988)

Love Songs to the Shadow

In the early 1990s, I was presenting at a sound symposium, and one presentation was to play the human form as an instrument to demonstrate the compositional formulas that a body reveals. I had the good fortune to collaborate with exceptionally conscious musicians who trusted this work and supported the process.

The title of the concert was "Love Songs to the Shadow." My "instrument" was a client and friend with uterine cancer. She was clothed and lay on a massage table. I placed colored silks on her body at different times in concert to match the emotional timbre and the force or shape of the tones her body revealed.

The musicians played and interpreted the colors. I vocalized the music revealed by Maureen's human form, Mike Vargas was on piano, Mark McCoin on percussion instruments, Michael Stanwood on didgeridoo, and Farrell Lowe was on stick guitar. I tuned her body with my voice and received the arrangement from her body, then the musicians supported and improvised.

We prepared for the performance by meditating together to ground, plug into, our own bodies. During the performance, our intention was to stay connected to one another. If one of us disconnected, or if we did not authentically perceive sounds or shapes that needed to be expressed, we would pause, gather, wait, and listen until we again were connected and present. It kept us honest and relaxed, trusting that we did not know and ensuring that our work was listening, not just making sounds to fill in space.

Many of the sounds were of a dissonant nature, and we could feel and hear a rumbling of disagreement from some uncomfortable members of the audience. This was not "healing music"! The resistance was palatable. An underlying belief and expectation were present that healing music was always melodic and harmonic.

In our concert, if one listened with an open mind and ear, one would note formulas, a math of sorts, taking place as we followed the sound print of this human form. There would be dissonance, harmonics, melody, conversations, and dialogs from different parts of the body's consciousness as they were expressed and integrated. To the best of our ability, we were composing a sound print of what this body wished to have expressed. But I am afraid that many ears were deaf to this at the time.

Dr. Valerie Hunt was scheduled to address the entire conference directly following our Sacred Sound performance. Dr. Hunt was a pioneering scientist who was the first to measure the human bioenergy fields in the laboratories of UCLA. She is responsible for researching and validating that touch, movement, frequency, and intention can and does change the molecular structures, the chemistry of a human form.

Dr. Hunt validated that a web of consciousness surrounds us and changes as the result of vibrational frequencies. Electromagnetic fields increase through intentional touch and alignment. One can occupy a variety of conscious awareness states simultaneously. Dr. Hunt is responsible for the recognition of pioneering modalities brought forth by Dr. Ida Rolf, Emilie Conrad, Judith Aston, Rosalyn Bruyere, and many others. We are deeply indebted to this gentle, wise soul for validating for us what were considered metaphysical miracles.

Dr. Hunt was presenting her research with cancer cells that day. She reported that when working with cancer, degenerative diseases, and tumors, one must use RED frequencies first—strong sounds and intentions—to STOP and/or slow down the disease growth, create boundaries, activate cellular attention, and wake up the healing cells to block the cancerous cells, then we can bring in the softer, calming frequency influences. Dr. Hunt affirmed our work that day and the precision of what we were doing through sound.

I find that the dissonant sound is paramount to all work done with sound and color. I am always working in bipolar or tripolar frequency patterns, never in just one tonal category. There always seems to be the need for at least three, if not five or seven, ingredients in sound work to match the frequency, shape, and nutrition that the body is wanting. "A little red, then a bit of yellow, now green, catch that end with red, now smooth with blue."

Remember: sound *is* color, and by staying present we can perceive a colorful palette of listening. There are many functions served by dissonance sounds.

Often dissonance can be the most challenging sounds to get our clients to vocalize. It is also challenging for people to make these sounds without hurting themselves by straining and stressing vocals or thinking that the sound must be loud; therefore, learning to soften the jaw is important.

The generic fear of expressing dissonance is fascinating and interesting with respect to belief systems of what a "good" sound is and what a "healing" sound is. There is magnified thinking in the human psyche about our fear of the shadow. I cannot help but believe our religions of the West are a big contributor to this fear. Unfortunately, what has been called the "new spirituality" seems to have embraced some of that ideology as well.

The Collective Shadow

During the last couple of years, the light has been cast quite loudly and painfully on the collective shadow within us all. After the 2016 Presidential election in the United States, my first thought was that few people on this planet could raise their hands and honestly say that we humans are not racist or sexist on a global level. I know this era is, and has been, a most challenging time—not only for the United States but for the entire world. It does seem to be shining light on the shadow. And for this I am grateful.

I need to look inside and see where my racism is, where my sexism is—not to shame myself but to become willing to be more honest and use sounding to empty and dissolve anything that does not serve or enhance evolutionary possibilities. This is a life work, I know.

Thirty to 40 years ago, in private practice, I noticed layers of racism in all beings, regardless of gender, age, race, culture. This was so unexpected! I thought I knew something about racism and who had it!

As I went deeper into this shaping, I started finding that at the root of racism was self-hatred in the physical form. As the self-hatred came up through the many layers of tissue to the outer realm of personality, it was and is lived and expressed as "hatred of the other." We know racism is thousands of years old, and here I have simplified something that is a most treacherous weaving throughout the innards of humanity. But sometimes, it is easier to unwind if I just keep it simple.

Can I practice self-loving as a means to embracing loving others? I need a daily practice of loving myself unconditionally, a willingness to dissolve and surrender old belief systems that keep me from loving. I am needing, desiring, to go toward love.

I cannot afford to hate. Hate hurts me as well as others. Hating is most toxic for my health and well-being. Hating is a thief of my life force. I may not be able to like everyone, but I cannot afford to hate them. I make amends by sounding, surrendering, and digesting old emotions and experiences. I move from the inward terrains to the outer living, as these inner changes show up in my relationships. It is important to honestly acknowledge that the body reveals where my "conditions of love" are living.

I was fortunate as a young woman to be near Dr. Martin Luther King and his teachings. His example of nonviolence, along with the teachings of Mahatma Gandhi decades earlier, revealed to me the power of love. They both recognized that hate would kill their spirit, their essence. It would kill the message their soul was here to impart. We learned to love by knowing how much we wanted to hate.

Sound All You Hate

Sound all you love.
Sound all you hate.
And sound all that you love again.
Begin and end with love.

Sound your gratitude.
Sound your grace.
Sound your self.
Awake!
Over and over again.

Life Magazine

Yeah, I made *Life* magazine, sometime in 1964 or '65. People would say, "Oh, I bet your Mama was proud." Well, you might say it got her busy. She went and bought up every *Life* magazine she could find in Southern Illinois, in Eastern Missouri, and part ways toward Louisville, Kentucky.

"Now doesn't that beat all!" exclaimed my liberal friend Diana, trying to act Southern. Yeah, "it beats" all alright. She bought them up so no one would see the picture of me demonstrating for Blacks to have the human right to vote!

That's how big her fear was chasing her back then. And that's how fast a cross could be burnt in your yard, and that's all she knew to do back then—to hide to protect her kin.

Sound Transforms the Blues to Gold

Sound transforms the blues to gold. Dissonance is an essential ingredient within a healing formula. I started sounding to stay alive. I continue sounding to stay vital, plugged in, stimulated, energized, cleared, and unstuck—to stay sane. The rhythms of dissonance create a stimulating pulse in the fluid system for reorganization and movement toward coherence.

The path of wellness may look like the path of discord as we follow it. Find the shape. Invite it home. Allow it to come into current time. Sound what is there. Bring the entire body along. Let your body be shaped by following the path of least resistance. Look for the soft spot. God comes through the wound.

Emotional Wound

> "To get to God, at the core of God at his greatest,
> one must first get into the core of himself at his least."
> ~ **Meister Eckhart,** theologian

When an emotional wound doesn't receive the mending needed for healing, it may become an energetic magnet that attracts other wounding to it. Our thoughts, feelings, sensitivities, and responses to life reflect the emotional wound. Often what is needed for mending is to be truly listened to without judgment. Much of the judgment comes from the self. Sounding provides a slowing down and perspective; it creates a rhythm for listening and mending, a layer at a time. We do not know the timing or the layer of the insertion or the root of the emotional wound.

We may not know how deeply we were affected or how much attention we may have needed. Or we may have acted like or believed that we did not need help, thus denying our innate wisdom and feeling/emotional body. Our body is waiting to be heard by a listening ear. Possible symptoms of denied expression of emotional wounding are:

- Every nuance is taken personally.
- There becomes self-centeredness that "all is about me."
- My wounding is interpreting and shaping my life experiences.
- The wounding starts layering physically and creating its own world of story.
- Everything bothers it, and we get really touchy.

Revealing What Is Not Mine

How do we heal this wounding? One layer at a time. We sound one layer of fascia at a time. The energetic pattern of the emotional wound lives in the tissue. The issues are in the tissues. We sound the top layer, the one that is right on the surface—no digging, no working, no figuring.

Sound what is just right there, what is effortless. We unwind emotional, undigested wounding on each layer with our voice. As we sound this top layer, it dissolves the story matter and is transformed into fluid and then the next layer comes to the surface and presents itself.

This is using sound as bodywork, a deep tissue work with accurate listening and respect for the intelligence of this human form. What is ready to be sounded for mending and integrating reveals itself to us. Just sound what is revealed to create a fluidity, to dissolve the "story" of that layer. It may not be the core of the wound, as the superficial tissues created several bandages of protection. It takes many layers to get to the core, but it keeps revealing itself and unraveling.

In the first layer, there is unwinding and unwrapping from one's daily living. These are often not our personal wounds. It is very easy for us to gather fragments from the thoughts of others, from the feelings of others, and layer these into our internal environment, and call it "us." This is often the first layer we sound; we are emptying what is not ours, then we can start seeing what is needed. The body starts revealing what is there and the sound solution.

Loving Self-Care Made Simple

Our vocalizing can be very helpful as we sound one layer of tissue at a time in order to unwind emotional, undigested wounding. Just sound what is revealed in order to create a fluidity, to dissolve the "story" of that layer. At the superficial layer, as noted, these are not our personal wounds; they are collections from our daily life. It is easy to gather fragments from the thoughts and feelings of others and layer these environments upon ourselves.

This is what needs to be emptied by sounding often. If we do not empty ourselves, we can start to identify with these energies; therefore, our intention with loving self-care is simple: to take personal responsibility for sounding and emptying our field regularly of those things that are not ours. This relieves us of any judgments we have about other people's stuff. The more we harmonize our field, the more protected and calm we feel.

Sounding these superficial layers is "sounding what is not ours." To put it simply, it is a given that we are always exchanging energy with all humanity, all the time. It's not a wrong thing to do; it simply is occurring. We don't even need to know what is not ours. What is most important to understand is that we cannot heal, mend, or integrate what is not ours!

The Accuracy of Sound as Bodywork

For those of you who are bodyworkers, massage therapists, Rolfers, tissue workers by any name, I wish to impart what I have learned from working the tissue with sound, listening, presence, and intention.

As mentioned at the beginning of this book, when I was studying myofascial technique in the 1970s, I discovered that sound could change the tissue. As I applied voice to the area of concern, sound started teaching me what it knew, which was finding the direction the tissue needed to unwind and release.

I witnessed sound literally hydrating the tissue and increasing the volume of dimension to the musculature. Sound rearranged and reorganized the tissue in its most supportive way. Through these many years that I have been practicing sound as bodywork, I combined it with hands-on bodywork, as my clients were not sure if sound alone could give them what they needed. That was before all my clients became remote during the pandemic time. We discovered that sound alone does the work that is needed.

As noted, deep tissue work begins by sounding the superficial layers that take us to the deeper layers. We always start at the layer or layers presenting. Our sounding hydrates that layer and allows the layer to be restored and returned to its liquid state. Sound changes the tissues, the alignment, and the structure of the body. We are always working with the intelligence of the body.

Wounding and injury dehydrates our tissues.
Sounding hydrates our tissues.
Sound restores three-dimensionality at a cellular level.

Our bodies are intricate tapestries of weavings. This tapestry consists of fascia, tendons, muscles, nerve fibers, blood, cells, and bone—all the ingredients that make up the physiology of our physical terrain—and it is repeated layer after layer.

If we sound the layer that is presenting, any holding within that layer begins to dissolve, rest, and regain elasticity. The next layer then arises and presents itself. By intentionally working one layer at a time, we help bring the body to a place of integration.

The accuracy comes from the wisdom of the body and us being able and willing to trust this innate wisdom. If I voice what is revealing itself and not try to change or rearrange, fix it, or heal it, if I follow the body's direction, it will organize itself in a most coherent and cohesive way. This is a deep, spiritual trust. It has taken me decades to get the feel and texture of trust. I get a glimpse, a glimmer of what "rest assured" means at the deeper layers.

I need to stay out of the way of the intelligence of resonance. Our sounds are expressing the "imprints," the holding patterns, the injuries, and belief systems, as we "unwind" a layer at a time.

We are listening for the blueprint and encoding within the body. We are sounding and dissolving the holding patterns of the imprints in the body's tissue. Our intention is to perceive and be restored to the resonance of our inherent "blueprint," the soul's purpose and original template.

Often these wounded, undigested places get stuck in chronological time within the tissue. Unexpressed, stored emotions literally shape and distort our perceptions of the world and hinder and restrict our own flow of liquid health. I don't need to know or have an interpretation of what that means.

Many interpretations are floating around the collective energy field and are magnetically attracted by a frequency that matches the initial wounding. Our sounding can dissolve the layered energies that have become magnetically attached to what we have been calling "ours." Simply sound what the body is revealing.

Allowing the Body to Get to Current Time

When the infrastructure of magnetized layering can be dissolved,
there is the possibility of revealing the layer of insertion of the wound.
Allow the sound and wisdom of the wound
to unwind itself to current time,
to come home to now.

This is the gift of sounding ourselves over and over. Sound dissolves unexpressed layers and restores and nourishes the emotional body. Sound is one of our finer tools for healing emotionally. We can assist our emotional body as it matures, integrates, and assimilates a layer at a time.

In our deeper research, we find many young emotional memories embedded in our tissue. Sounding a layer at a time, we bring that younger place into current time. Weaving a thread at a time, the tapestry is mended. We come home to now.

Remember, we are returning to the concept of "matching." If I match the emotional feeling body, with the rhythms and tonal color of what I am perceiving, the alchemy of transformation takes place. I am not trying to change or fix. I am meeting, matching, what is there, and the intelligence of my inner wisdom does the transformation.

When we start sounding the nuances of interpretations, they often sound dissonant—sad moans or cries or painful tears—as noted earlier on. But sound as bodywork is precise and efficient. If I sound the first layer, it dissolves and becomes more liquid, allowing the next layer to bubble up to the surface and reveal itself. It then becomes the superficial layer that has our attention. You get to the deeper layers by working with one superficial layer at a time. This is a practice. For me, it is a life work. The layers are infinite and glorious to be recognized as our true nature becomes more evident with time and practice.

Key Points for Sounding Multiple Layers

- With our voices, we invite an awakening of the potential to arrive at a layer of current timing. We are voicing the sounds, expressions, colors, and shapes of all these stored feelings, real or imagined.

143

- We are sounding denied feelings of wounding, allowing them to come to current time. We are voicing these sounds to awaken our rhythms and the pulse of vitality in our various systems.
- We acknowledge each layer as we seek integrated healing, while we travel deeper into the pathway of our wounding.
- We refrain from a tendency to dig or dive into the layer of insertion. As we have stated earlier, we do not tear tissue sonically to get results. We respect the body's wisdom of uncovering and revealing itself when it is ready to do so.
- We become more accurate as we practice listening and observing what is and what is possibly not ours within our bodies.
- The body's homeostasis is rearranged each time we sound, and we need to give time, even days, to experience the new balance of support the body wishes to reveal and experience.
- Our voices can and do touch and reflect the many layers and variables that the body is showing. Through our listening voice, we can register and express the emotions, the full range of the many diverse voices within.
- Instruments, such as tuning forks, singing bowls, and drums, add another dimension emotionally and spiritually, and complement integration.

We are listening for the blueprint and encoding within the body. We are sounding and dissolving the holding patterns of the imprints in the body's tissues. Our intention is to perceive and to be restored to the resonance of our inherent blueprint, the soul's purpose and original template.

Harmonics to Dissonance

All I have learned in this life is that dissonance lives in the harmonics and harmonics live in the dissonance. If I follow the dissonant sounds and tones and rest in them, they will turn into a beautiful, harmonic, tonal quality. This is the means of allowing the wounding to come into current time—letting dissonance live in harmonics, and harmonics live in dissonance. Many of us love harmonic overtone singing. Listen closely, and you will hear how the overtones originate from a dissonant sound, a nasal pitch, or a deep belly and throat sound.

What is Your Form of Perceiving?

- Own and acknowledge how you perceive.
- What do you know about yourself and how you perceive?
- What are your natural gifts?
- What can you rely on?
- What is your "knowing"?
- People have various ways of perceiving. It is important that you practice and trust your own instincts and experience.
- Some perceive through energetics of touch, of vision, of voice, of scent.
- Others perceive through color, shapes, and geometries.
- Some through a felt sense within the body.
- What are your preferences?

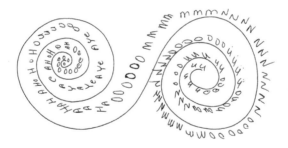

Formulas for the Emotional Body

A formula refers to the way we are addressing all the bodies, all the characters. It means we find different components on any given layer, as we are seeking the rhythm of that body. Below are some examples of formulas we could use for someone who is in a lot of fear or suffering from trauma or abuse. Often, I will be working with three elements in a formula; for instance, color components, frequency, and intention.

There is no such a thing as a "healing" sound. All sounds are healing, at the right time, for the right person, in the right place.

1. The Soothing Formula

This is a comforting sound in nearly any language or culture. Parents and families have been soothing upsets and restlessness with each other for thousands of years with "*Shhhh . . .* it's alright; *shhhh . . .* rest now—you are safe." *Shhh* is not an admonishment of "*Shush*, be quiet!" It is soothing: "*Shhhh . . .* rest assured. You are safe."

Soothing is so important, as it helps all the bodies (physically, emotionally, mentally, spiritually) to settle down, to let go of tension from a myriad of reasons, and the variety and relationships of characters and ages within the psyche.

I have spent entire sessions using variations of this soothing sound. Knowing of course that every situation is unique, so the circumstances and the impact of soothing sound varies with each person. The following example is of great value.

CLIENT SESSION
Healing Deep Trauma

I recall a most brutal situation of a party gang rape for a young woman who came to me for healing. Her body was frozen. Her emotions were threads of fear, remorse, guilt, shame, blame, and confusion. I am sure you know or have heard how often the abused person feels guilt and blames themselves for having caused and received the abuse. We know there are many cultural historic reasons that create this traumatic response.

She was a being in deep pain. She lay on the table fully clothed and covered with a blanket. As she could not allow touch, I did not touch her at all during our first sessions, nor for the longest time. I stood 3 to 4 feet away and sounded her body with love song energies interspersed with lullabies. As she cried and cried and moaned her pain, I started moaning and making crying sounds with her.

I was trying to match her frequencies as well as I could. My intention was to give a soundscape in an unintrusive way so she would not feel self-conscious discomfort and could just make any sounds she needed as I held the space in sounds that matched hers.

As I honored the safe distance her body needed, I walked around to the foot of the table or to her other side. After a while, her releasing started slowing down and quieting, I started Humming and *Shhhing*, Humming and *Shhhing*.

At first, I began quite loudly, then slowly got quieter, at which point I started walking closer to the table, Humming and Shhhing for the rest of session. When I knew she could hear me in terms of listening to a directive, I suggested that she Hum or *Shhhh* to herself softly. I also invited her, as comfort allowed, to place her hands on her heart area while *Shhhing*. We ended that session with her learning to soothe herself with Hum and *Shhh* soundings.

This is not a "quick fix." Traumatic happenings are never such, but we had the opportunity to experience a few more sessions. Having tools of sound, her own touch, and visualization, a spiritual connection could be rekindled within her. It all takes time, sometimes an entire lifetime.

I did not know what she needed, so I waited for her body to give me the clues. I started with love; universal love, let's call it. Then she started directing, and I followed. When a person is in deep trauma, we move slowly within their auric field space. We move in soft arc-shaping, spiral, curved motions. My focus and intention were to touch the layer that could assist to call her home.

Again, I always return to our Hum Signature, as it has the ingredients to restore fragments that have been detached by accidents, deep grief, inhumane treatment, and so forth. Perhaps that body cannot handle any more diversity of sounds beyond the Hum. It would be intrusive to go into a deeper and complex layer. First, allow this body to rest. From rest, the body will be available for what is next.

2. The Emptying Formula

Often what is labeled "emotion" is the noise within the mental body. I may be having a mental conversation with myself—noise in my head. By sounding the noise, I am dissolving the noisy fragments into fluidity. By sounding the noise, I become inwardly more quiet. Remember we are always sounding to be restored to liquid.

We can begin by listening, and asking: "Who or what is wanting to be attended to first?" What conversation, or inner character, needs to express? The loudest one? Possibly. Let's clear that out first, perhaps with aerobic sounds. The body will naturally reveal what is to follow.

HA HE HA HE. Syllabic sounds, aerobic sounding, and gibberish are all considered emptying sounds.

Then we find another voice, a different rhythm, and a different tone. *SHALA NOKA BYA DIKU . . .* All sounds arise spontaneously without you or me "thinking" them or deciding that a specific sound or syllabic sequence must be created. *SHALA NOKA BYA DIKU!*

Then, we hear another voice coming forward, likely with a different tone and rhythm.

OOOH SHU SHU NALA . . . OOOH SHU SHU NALA . . .

With sounding, all the various aspects and ages of ourselves have their say, express their sound signature. No analysis. We do not need to know why this sound is coming out of the body, how it got there, or what it means. We are simply letting everybody have a voice, in their own rhythm and time.

Sounds of the emotional body will often be dissonant. The emotions have a bad reputation—that releasing them will be extreme, bad. "Don't move that anger, because it will blow up the town." But by sounding, we discover that our system *wants* to express and integrate all the emotional colors and energy layers.

3. The Integrating Formula

We take what we've sounded and move them together to create integration. We want to weave all the threads and fibers of sound together. We have separated them to understand the fragments and characters. Then we integrate every bit of that layer. We are trying to bring all the fragments home through our integration formula. As a result of trauma, we separate or fragment; very lovingly, through our sounding practice, we work one layer at a time in order to mend and reweave.

The integration of those diverse threads hydrates the musculature. It creates a proportionate, dimensional reclaiming, and the body becomes more liquid. The expression of the emotions allows the tissue to hydrate and fill out dimensionally what was compressed or constricted.

We take the sounds we are working with and put them into a blender, mixing them up inside the cavernous shape of our mouth and throat until they spin and twist themselves into a tone, very much like how we took our name and turned it into our Hum. We gather our sounds into a spiral to integrate the diverse layers and character, inviting them to be included in their rightful position within our tissue.

HA HE HA KYA OKE TU UMMMMHUMMMMMMMMM SHSHSHSHSH.

As the words merge into sound, they become spiraling energy that weaves all those threads together and integrates every bit of that layer of our tapestry. We spin and twist to dissolve fragmentation.

Please note: The three approaches discussed here are not a protocol, a fixed formula, to heal trauma. They are simply a sounding example, where we touch various layers that are holding parts of the story and need and want to be dissolved and reintegrated into the whole. As we have found, often the parts that have been traumatized literally become fragments that break off and fall away from the body. Our focus is to bring these fragmented aspects of ourselves home. May I be in acceptance of all of me.

"Why do Yaminahua shamans talk in twisted language?
According to one of them:
'With my koshuiti I want to see—
singing, I carefully examine things—

149

twisted language brings me close but not too close—
with normal words, I would crash into things—
with twisted ones, I circle around them—
I can see clearly.'"

    ~ **Jeremy Narby,** anthropologist

I always speak of bringing the sound into a spin, into a spiral to integrate, to see, to explore our unseen world. I am very grateful and humbled to know that through the wisdom of sound current teachings and inner journeys, I stumbled into a terrain of listening as the ancient earth has taught so many on this planet. I understand so clearly what this Amazonian shaman is saying about words. I found the same. Words have edges; sound rounds the edges.

Decades ago, while working with people who had been abused with hurtful words from strong emotions of hate or humiliation, I noticed a special distinction: These layers of wounding were much harder to dissolve than the layers of abuse that came from being physically hit or kicked. Not to say one is less or more; just that the words get lodged within the tissue and are played over and over in the mind. Sounding in a spinning way dissolves the words and allows the person to receive what is most needed. Sound rounds the corners.

I am grateful that the quote by Jeremy Narby, author of *The Cosmic Serpent,* was recently brought to me. We all need affirmation of our innate wisdom. My hope and prayerful intentions are that these *Audible Body* writings will bring some affirmation to you, dear readers, of your own "knowing."

"Expression of emotions is a gateway to touching, igniting, and recognizing our mystic natures. The resonance that sounding produces with intention and with grounded presence creates a liquid electric environment which is conducive to the Soul's terrain."

    ~ **Dr. Valerie Hunt,** scientist

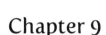

Chapter 9

Sound as a Spiritual Solution

"The magic of 'Musical Medicine' will come into its own. The application of such healing potencies will not be limited just to man's body and mind. It will be an agency for building and healing his soul as well."

~ **Corinne Heline,** Christian mystic

Bali: Sing a Love Song to Your Shadow

The time I spent in Bali, many years ago, brought about some of my deeper teachings of learning to love unconditionally. In Bali, all the sacred forms—dance, music, theater, and religious practices—are a daily ritual of honoring the shadow and the light.

The qualities of good and evil are given equal honor and homage. Every day each household, business, and neighborhood prepares altars of fruit, incense, and flowers for their good and evil deities.

This was truly life-changing. Until then, I had been teaching how to sound and rid oneself of the evil, the shadow. All we wanted was light, so we continually emptied with sound what was dark or considered impure, and uncomfortable. If only we thought more positively, we would be alright, and our shadow, or evil, would eventually vanish. My belief system was that if I starve the shadow self, ignore it, deny it, shame it, feel guilty about it, and blame it, the shadow self will go away!

Bali cracked open my limited range. One evening while visiting the home of a Hindu priest, I noticed that his altars were paying homage to both good and evil.

I asked, "Why do you feed that which you call evil?"

He said: "One night an evil spirit is walking down my street and sees my home and thinks, *That looks like a good place to live.* But my evil deity, which I have been feeding and caring for these many years, is now my protector. He says, 'You keep going spirit. This is my home.' He protects me; he is my ally."

I was beginning to get a crack in my deep belief system.

Balinese culture believes that one cannot have light without dark. What a revelation. I had thought that I understood this, but seeing it lived out daily, it came in and softened and rounded my corners more and more. I had been trying to starve my shadow to death, literally. And as we discover, over and over, that which is repressed or ignored only gets stronger. In the early 1970s, sound had taught me that what is unexpressed runs the show. Ah, some belief systems have deeper roots than we know.

My suggestion right now is this: If you have a Source, a God, that you are not good enough for, you may want to consider getting a Source that loves you unconditionally. It's allowed.

What a gift. As I was preparing to leave Bali, I asked the deities of the spirit and earth: "What will I do when I return home? I cannot set out food where I live daily. Mountain lions will be attracted to my house [in those years, I lived in the foothills of the Rocky Mountains]. How can I honor my light and my dark?"

Here were the instructions given me by the nature spirits of that place on Earth:

Sing daily a love song to my shadow.
Sing a love song to that which I fear this day.
A love song for what I am judging.
A love song for what I fear is not good enough,
or wise enough, or hasn't done enough.
I sing a love song to exactly how I am that moment daily,
regardless of my situation, real or imagined.

Key Points for Singing a Love Song to Shadow

- Remember, this is good medicine!
- Practicing unconditional love is a daily inside job.
- Teach me how to unconditionally love myself; I do not know how.
- May I learn to love myself unconditionally.
- Teach me how to unconditionally love others; I do not know how.
- Teach me to be willing to love myself unconditionally.
- I am grateful I am willing to love unconditionally.

This daily prayer revealed how many conditions I had about loving myself and loving others. If I cannot accept my own human frailty, I cannot accept yours.

EXERCISE
Singing a Love Song to Ourselves

Beauty is needed in times of stress. There are times when our bodies very much need the beauty of a love song. Most days singing a love song to ourselves is a helpful, restorative, stress releasing, comforting, responsible act of kindness.

- Start with the Hum.
- Listen deeply to the love that wants and needs to be expressed.
- Give it your voice, and breathe in this love, and breathe out this love in your song, in your sound.
- We are sounding to get the mind out of the way. We are sounding to remove some of the power from the upper brain and spread the circuitry of wisdom to the lower brain, and eventually to the heart brain, for yet greater understanding, vision, and acceptance.
- Sound gets the mind out of the position of being the authority over the body. The mind has been protecting us and we are grateful, but we are going to a greater authority. We are going to our soul for guidance and direction for our growth.

Loving Our Many Characters

"Your task is not to seek for love, but merely to seek and find all the barriers within yourself that you have built against it."

~ **Rumi,** Sufi mystic

Every age we have ever been, and possibly every age we will become, is recorded in our body. We observe the interplay of various characters and ages within us communicating. We communicate and engage these characters in sound formulas.

The first archetype I suggest you work with is your inner guide, teacher, sage, the wise one in you, the one that absolutely has your best interests at heart and loves you unconditionally.

Find that character. Start a conversation, a relationship, with this being. This is a practice of trusting. It is an acceptance that you do have an inner guide, teacher. Spending time in inquiry with this guiding aspect of self is foundational work. Developing a relationship with one that protects you and always has your best interests at heart is truly helpful when you invite other aspects of self into the formula.

Here is a list of possible archetypical characters. I invite you to add your own:

The wise one	The teacher	The procrastinator
The healer	The victim	The guilty one
The good parent	The good child	The angry one
The bad parent	The bad child	The dictator
The people pleaser	The fearful one	The doubter
The belligerent one	The rejected one	The misunderstood one
The brat	The superior one	

Do you get the idea? Do you identify with any of these characters? Please make your own list of characters you can identify with.

Now we look at a formula concept pertaining to these characters. As our intention is to create communication, we want to open a dialog between our various voices and attitudes.

Many times, it can seem like an inner battle of many feuds or a placement of who has the biggest voice or presence. Some of these characters may never fully like one another, but they can learn to become willing to cooperate or to be teachers and healers for one another. In this context, we can call on certain inner characters for certain tasks. Simply let everybody have a voice in their own rhythm and time.

My spiritual teaching and intention for myself is to cease the inner battle, cease the fighting among my many aspects. I want to invite cooperation, invite dialog, and invite cohesiveness within my entire body. The desire is to be in good relationship with all parts of self.

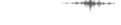

EXERCISE
Ask Your Inner Characters

- What is your rhythm?
- What is your color?
- What do you want to say or express?
- What do you need me to know?

For example, I choose to communicate with the Procrastinator and the Victim, and My Wise One, My Teacher. I will do an inquiry with each, telling them that I want to know them better. I want to know what their needs are, and I want to understand how to have better communication and cooperation with each of them.

That in a sense is the inquiry. Primarily, the message is that I sincerely want to hear what each character must say, and I will do my research with sound and movement. I will let myself voice each character and then I will pause and listen. (Please refer to chapter 1 for the more in-depth self-inquiry.)

I need and want to write, but I don't write, and then I feel guilty and victimized because I am not doing so. I go back and forth between feeling the presence of the desire, the guilt, and the victim.

A vicious circle creates more not-doing.

I need to call my Teacher/Inner Guide into this group to shine some light upon the patterns of these characters in order to decrease the blame and shame and see what is needed for these aspects of self to be willing to take some action.

Now during this scenario/session arrives yet another character, a different voice. Let's call it the Passionate One, the Writer, the Artist. Greatly needed in this conversation, they create an opening and an understanding. This allows the Victim and the Guilty character to relax and listen to what can serve the whole, what serves my desire and need to write. To do that, I need help and willingness and passion from all aspects of myself to be present.

By adding the Passionate Writer and Artist to this sound inquiry, I am given a completely different experience than I thought I was after. My inner knowing once again shows me the wisdom of what is needed for this healing. What brings relief, insight, or cooperation from this vicious circle is to allow other perspectives. Let us hear from the Artist in me. Let sound do the teaching, the mending, the knowing. I begin with a premise and stay willing to have it change. My beginning is just that, a place to start—a way into this inner terrain, this galaxy of possibilities. Sound is a transformational tool.

Process for Loving Our Many Characters

- I have a desire, an intention to know and understand each inner aspect, and to learn how these characters can live more cooperatively together. I do not know the outcome; I trust the process of pausing, listening, loving, intending, emptying, whining, and blending the characters' stories.

- I could begin with words. I am not sure who is coming first, possibly Victim. Victim's words might be, "I never do what I want. I can't, and I'm too tired." Sounds a lot like Procrastinator, ummm? "We will write after we call Sonja."

- I whine and complain and turn the words into sounds, get the story out of the words. The sounds have the intention, the conversation, the emotional psychological shaping of my movements. Walking, turning, breathing—each has its own rhythms. Take the words away.

- Sound creates a curve, rounds the corners of the words, and allows them to spin into coherence, putting a twist, a spin on the sounds to integrate the expression into fluidity.
- The Wise Teacher is here observing without judgment, holding the space of listening, letting the characters sound until they tire a bit of their "rightness."
- Then the Passionate Artist appears in their unquestionable desire to create with the knowingness that it is possible. Now colors of hope spring forth as unification becomes more important to the whole.

The voices of the characters get to express without receiving any judgment. Just by being heard they often let go of their position of being right. The emotion or position starts dissolving, resolving, and cooperation begins. When we feel completely listened to our story starts dissolving. We do not need it fixed or therapized. Our deep desire is to be restored to our essence, which is liquid.

We learn to respect our own timing of characters with acceptance and gratitude. We discover our bodies are willing to communicate and that we are willing to listen to the complexity of the languages within our internal tapestry. Spending time listening to our own characters is important before we begin to listen to the complex math of unwinding the wounding of others.

Let the sound have its way. Let the characters have their say.

When they feel completely listened to their story starts dissolving.

Our purpose in sounding is to be restored to our essence,
which is liquid.

Sometimes we make masks or drawings of our different characters. Sometimes it is helpful to make a drawing or representation of what we heard during a sounding session. Consider these questions as part of noting your session formulas. These are just suggestions:

- What percentage of space does each character occupy?
- What percentage of time did each character sound?
- What colors or movements happened during the session?
- What was the sensation when cooperation began and the characters came together?
- What expression did the characters need before they felt heard?
- Which characters really helped bring about a solution or integration?
- What helps you remember and track what happens in your laboratory?
- Perhaps you can also notice where the sensations are in the body?

EXERCISE
Character Formula Laboratory

- Follow the pathway of your own inquiry, in your own laboratory of rhythm.
- Journal the sound bites or expressions of the archetypes you perceive.
- Listen. Which rhythm comes first? Second?
- Follow the order of rhythm.
- Follow pathways of release, of wound, of health.
- Follow the pathway where the body is directing you to go.
- Journal the sound archetypes that you perceive.

We do not know the formula until the body reveals it to us. Once we enter this terrain of study with respect, the sound frequency reveals the pathway of one's healing. As we surrender, sound takes us as its student. Sound frequency becomes our therapist. For example, here are drawings of the formulas I made during sounding training:

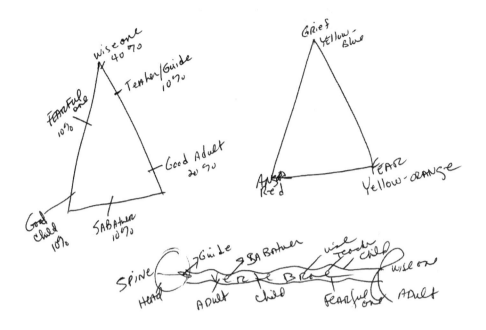

"We do not grow absolutely, chronologically.
We grow sometimes in one dimension, and not in another; unevenly.
We grow partially. We are relative.
We are mature in one realm, childish in another.
The past, present, and future mingle and pull us backward, forward, or
fix us in the present. We are made up of layers, cells, constellations."

~ **Anais Nin**, writer

The Spiritual Significance of Music

"Every illness is a musical problem—the healing, a musical solution."

~ **Novalis,** poet

I was once asked to write on what I believe is the spiritual significance of
music. Sound has the power to awaken me and remind me what is truly
important, and what follows is my response:

SOUND stirs my blood, deepens my breath, quiets my mind,
caresses my trust, cultivates my passion, restores me to "right size,"
reminds me to move, reminds me that I am movement,
reminds me that I love to move,
reminds me that I am ageless,
reminds me of times past that moved me to tears, to joy, to the depths
of grief, to clarity of NOW,
to remember, yes, to remember that I am connected to something greater.
Yes, I AM . . . Oh, thank you.
My heart and belly sings, I had forgotten again . . .

And you Sound, you Strings, you Heartbeat, you Rhythm,
you Dissonance, match my fabric, my form.
Sonic light, you beam me free again, each time, you never fail,
to awaken me to what is real,
what is important,
and you always teach me to let go of that which is burdening me,
you always help me to empty my vessel
that I may have room for love and hope and compassion for this living . . .
you **SOUND**, you **MUSIC,**
remain my teacher and guide.

You teach me to follow the path through my blood,
through my nervous system,
You teach me to listen,
but mainly you show me over and over
that this is the path of over and over,
to forget and to remember and to forget and to remember . . .
and that you **SOUND,**
have the power of alchemy
to change that which has become coagulated in my liquid form
to be restored to an elixir of Ease . . .

For this I am grateful,
each time I come to you.

The Power of Sound and Vibration Being Made Visible

I was invited to be a lecturer at the 1999 Cortona Week in Cortona, Italy. This was a weeklong residential conference bringing together eminent physicists, scientists, artists, and philosophers from all over the world in a monastery turned hotel. The speakers and attendees were focused on radical transformative learning.

I saw that Dr. Hortensia ("Stan") Reintjens-Anwari had personally recommended me. My dear friend Stan was a worldly scholar whom I met in 1970 when I rented a room in her apartment in Cologne, Germany. I could not have been more surprised that our connection from decades earlier was bringing me this experience.

Dr. Luis Luigi, chair of the ETH Chemistry and Material Science departments in Zurich, founded these annual Cortona Week events in 1985. The gathering was held at this old monastery, on olive tree-graced grounds, within the closed Etruscan city of Cortona. Dr. Luigi wanted his Ph.D. students to be exposed to a diverse and expanded vision of the world. Each year his team created a theme—this year's was Creation.

Upon entering the olive tree gardens of the aged monastery, we were graciously received by Brother David Steindl-Rast, a world-renowned Benedictine monk, teacher, and author who meditates and writes on "the gentle power of gratefulness." Brother David, now in his late 90s, is committed to interfaith dialogue and the interaction between spirituality and science. He was invited every year and held spiritual grace and calm for all who attended.

I was to present my lecture mid-week, which afforded me the opportunity to observe and listen to several lectures before I was to give my presentation. This group of scholars was not like the touchy-feely groups I interacted with in such places as Esalen Institute on the Big Sur coast of northern California. These lecturers were physicists from Italy, Germany, France, England, the United States, China, and Switzerland. I found it most interesting that all lectures and classes were spoken in English, as that is the language of science, but it was the second or third language of most presenters and participants. Our group numbered about 400.

I quickly grasped that I had best not speak my esoteric-metaphysical science mind, that my humor could easily be misunderstood and cause confusion, and my esoteric mathematician self would be eaten for lunch.

Umm... what was I to do? I could find no words for an outline and was unable to prepare my presentation. I was supposed to speak for two hours about the transformational power of sound, yet when I turned inward to retrieve what I lived fully and knew so well, my mind was blank and became more blank, and I became more fearful each day.

This was my worst nightmare! I walked. I prayed on my knees, on my belly. I sat in meditation. I begged my Source for help. Fear had me paralyzed. Surrender was my only action. I prayed and I meditated some more. I knew nothing, and nothing was coming.

The day arrived for my two-hour lecture on Creation. It would be followed by a 15-minute Q&A and that truly petrified me! During other speakers' Q&A segments I had witnessed the massacre of critiques take place! Each lecturer was challenged harshly to defend their premise and theory.

Approaching the podium, I tell you again in most sincere honesty, I had nothing prepared, I had nothing to say. I was blank. I was reconciled to apologize to the organization and say, "I am unable to present," but upon facing the audience I opened my mouth, and this came out:

Ya me se me lo me se la te me Masa la me lo me la se me Mo te la se me lo

te ma

Si la ma lo mo ma lo

Te ke ka la so ma

Mi te la so fa

Me ke la te

Me la so

Te la me

This sound prayer flowed out of my mouth into the room for about 10 minutes. Like a purple silk ribbon, its graceful rhythms and tones created a huge pyramid shape of purple/violet that floated above the audience, then slowly descended, and enveloped all of us. People in the audience moved closer together, put their arms around one another, affectionately. Some were touched so deeply they cried.

When the prayer ended, I spoke to the audience about the grandmas and grandpas I was raised around and the trees and plants that were my first teachers and language. I was totally honest about my story, coming from the ridge of the Ozarks, an area completely removed from academic teachings.

I was compelled to invite a woman from the audience to join me on stage so that I could give her a sound session as a demonstration. She accepted, and we padded a table with some shawls for her comfort. I sounded her spine in the same way I attend all my clients, and the demonstration was no longer than 10 minutes. Later, someone informed me that during the previous days this woman had been very disruptive while interacting with many conference participants, and a lot of people had bad feelings toward her. I was also told that after receiving the sound demonstration from me, the woman became a more cooperative and compatible conference participant!

Coming out of the glow of the altered and protected state I had been in for the past couple of hours, I braced myself for the Q&A segment. I was very vulnerable. I knew I had no defense except Source.

A gentleman stood up, way in the back of the room, Dr. Tu. He commenced to describe all that I had done from his perspective of ancient Chinese philosophy, medicine, and science. Dr. Tu was very influential as an interface between the Dalai Lama and China, so his scientific description of my entire presentation was agreeable to the members of science who were present. He spoke in their language.

I do wish Dr. Tu's account had been recorded. I could not repeat, even moments after, the commentary he had so generously offered. I only heard acceptance, appreciation, and acknowledgment of these ancient teachings and of the arranging and rearranging of molecular form evidenced in the body in relation to the power of sound.

Dr. Tu provided a bridge and gave permission for these world-renowned physicists and artists to truly receive and honestly honor the emotional and spiritual depth they had experienced. Many participants expressed their gratitude to me for their experience. They had moved beyond theory.

I left the podium and went back to my room and sobbed with gratitude. *Thank you for removing the need of my personality to be something I wasn't and for giving me the courage to be what I am.* I was giving thanks to the mystery of us all.

I am grateful that there are people still alive who were there that day, who witnessed the power of mystery, the power of sound and vibration being made visible. The gift I was given was immense for this being. Never again did I need to defend or apologize for my perceptions.

Sound is the essence of creation.
Sound is the pulse, the impulse that resides in all living matter.
Sound makes visible the blueprint of our pathways.
May you find that now.

The Mythology of Awakening the Feminine Divine

Once upon a time, a very long time ago—several thousand years, for sure—the matriarchal age, the time of the Feminine Divine, was being dissolved for the Masculine Divine to enter.

The age change from matriarchy to patriarchy was taking place. Maybe similar, but not too dissimilar, to the times we are living in now. Now the patriarch is being transformed and removed to allow for the next phase of our evolution.

The last transformation was quite confusing for the inhabitants, as it is now. Much was unknown about what would prevail. There were many questions and fears about why there was a need for such radical change for the earth's inhabitants, not so unlike now.

There was and is much fear of the unknown, as now. I recall much concern our ancestors had for the loss of memory of the knowledge of nature, not unlike now.

Possibly the amnesia of not remembering was caused by the pure raw fear of the unknown, fear of changing the familiar. And a huge change it was to leave one's age of thousands of years to enter an unknown time for a new era, not unlike now.

It is reasonable that so much memory was lost and so much amnesia of events took place. Even though I cannot recall much of those times in any direct knowing, I do retain the frequencies of the earlier days and the progression of amnesia in the later days, very much like now.

The pain and the panic, the fear of the unknown; the fear of change, not unlike these days; the biological and emotional desire to stay alive—the Councils for Transitional Times had prophesized these events several hundred years prior to this time.

We were still not prepared for how quickly we would not know Source directly within our bodies, or the land we stood upon, or within the sunsets and the moon. Ah, and that the human form would not be honored as a holy vessel of rich tapestries of knowledge.

We reach into the ethers and feel how this may have been for those that had the sight of knowing what was coming. The wise ones knew that we are adaptogens, and we will adapt and we will forget, as now.

The Logistic Goddess Council made plans for the time when the memory of us beings would be awakened again to this sacred knowledge of the Feminine, and they declared that the memory of the future would be imprinted as "Encodements" within the physical form. They knew the safest place to hide wisdom was deep inside the human form, for the body is aligned with the earth itself. And I remember that being stated and sanctioned:

The blueprint "Encodements" will be safe here in the physical form, as no one will ever look deep into this sacred Temple to remember. Our memory of the Feminine Divine will stow away into the human physical form. They will not find us here, within the body.

The new times came. Most patriarchal religions all agreed that nature would not be included in the religion, and there would be only one God and that God would be male, and that male God would live outside the human realm, somewhere in the skies.

For thousands of years now, the human body has been considered less than spiritual, less important than the mind or the spirit; that to have enlightenment, one must leave this form, must deny this body.

I am of course shortening tens of thousands of years of interpretations. This is to give us a conversation to inspire a memory of possibly how much is denied and forgotten of our own nature. Many people were ridiculed for their culture's honorable ways and killed for remembering that we are nature. Not too different from these days yet, where accepting our own nature makes us still uncomfortable.

But this fragment of memory will birth more when it becomes necessary—the story goes on as I recall some of the fragments, real or imagined. I trust that possibly you remember parts of the story, before we forgot to remember. One day we may be blessed to share and put our memories together.

For those of us who have remembered through the many ages in a variety of forms, we are here now to listen to the "Encodements" within our bodies, to awaken the memory of our nature. The mythology has been to trust that the future time will bring equality of the male and female in all of us, and that we will be able and willing to cooperate in unity.

This we are telling our great-great-grandchildren, who are now preparing their entry.

May we retain memory, awaken memory. And may you, at your birthing, awaken a time of unification and knowing that we are a loving planet.

Appendix I

Additional Sound Vocabulary

Color-Sound Qualities

Color	Sound	Emotional Qualities Spectrum	
Red	E like in the word BE	Will & power activity. Freedom, determination, honor, will power, confusion, rebellion, strength, pioneer, consciousness, feeling, inspiration, motivation. catalyst.	Anger, authoritarianism, lust, frustration, force, confusion, violence, destruction, revenge, rebellion, impulsive, impatient, vengeance.
Blue	O like in the word NO	Love, wisdom, gentleness, trust, understanding, detachment, mercy, kindness, compassion, patience, forgiveness, cooperation, melody, contemplation, sensitivity, emotional security.	Possessiveness, self-pity, fear, self-rejection, indifference, separateness, isolation, worry, depression, passivity, anxiety, coldness, insecurity.
Yellow	ĂH like in the word AWE	Joy, expression, ability, mental discrimination, organization, attention to detail, evaluation, active intelligence, discipline, administration, praise, sincerity.	Criticism, crystallization, lazy, overindulgence, stubborn, constriction, contempt, sadness, selfish, cowardice, judgmental.
Green	AY like in the word SAY	All qualities of yellow and blue exist in green, plus: enthusiasm, energy flow, harmony, responsiveness, acceptance, hope, industrious effort, experience, gratitude, sharing, sustenance, expansion.	All qualities of yellow and blue exist in green, plus: jealousy, regimentation, envy, stinginess, pessimism, disorder, resistance, greed, resistance to harmony.

Color	Sound	Emotional Qualities Spectrum	
Orange	Ĕ like in the word LET	All qualities of yellow and red exist in orange, plus: illumination, courage, action, analysis, steadfastness, victory, confidence, intellect, harvest, interaction, change, striving, creativity, liberty, and freedom from force.	All qualities of yellow and red exist in orange, plus: uncooperativeness, inventiveness, sluggishness, inferiority, cruelty, superiority, pompousness.
Purple/ Violet	OU like in the word YOU	All qualities of blue and red exist in purple/violet, plus: self-motivation, service, responsibility, devotion, loyalty, understanding of justice, royalty, idealism, devotion & responsibility to leadership.	All qualities of blue and red exist in purple/ violet, plus: obsession, injustice, martyrdom, restriction, morose, intolerant, agitation, punishment.
Indigo	OM like in the word HOME	Synthesis, inspiration, ritual, ceremonial magic, implementation, persuasion, creativity, catalyst, aspirant, motivation, unity, calm, reminiscence.	Pride, separateness, conceit, arrogance, contempt, resentment, totalitarianism, irritability, gossip, rigidity.

Sound Formulas with Specific Interest

These are some suggestions and examples of geometry and directional possibilities with sounding. These are not facts, nor should you "marry" them. Consider them a bit of exploration for your creative nature. These also help us to remove linear sounding.

EE – Lateral.

AH – Open diagonally and laterally outward.

Jzzz – Softer, this creates more liquid in bone.

ZZ – Makes small mending movements at spine in all directions to the feed lines of the nervous system, expansive makes more liquid.

O – Vertical and rounded, expansive, creates groundedness as it extends.

a – Inside along spine, creates cushion, opening, diagonally inside.

u – Spirals, creating roundness inside.

e – Breaks up stuck, emotional places, chips away.

Appendix 2

Dr. Joseph Liss

Dr. Joseph Liss was one of my first mentors. He was hugely influential during my foundational years, and I want to acknowledge his influence on so many of us. I met him when I was a young hippy in the mid-1960s wanting to heal the world. Dr. Liss was a chiropractor and naturopathic doctor, herbalist, musician, poet, and a very wise philosopher. His store on Devon Avenue in Chicago comprised four walls of herbs, nuts, beans, dried fruits, cell salts, and a variety of staples. His clinic maintained three small cubicles, each with a small cot, table, and chair. He'd practiced there for 35 years, except in the 1940s, when he was imprisoned for five years for curing cancer without a medical license.

You may recall that psychoanalyst Wilhelm Reich was imprisoned and died as the result of his controversial Orgone theory, which stated that the molecular structure of the cancer cell could be modified. Dr. Liss had created an Orgone blanket, and both men had a similar vision, although they had never met or known one another. These stellar pioneers knew that combining various materials created an atmosphere of regeneration to change molecular structure.

Dr. Liss was ardent about the benefits of fasting, a cleansing diet, adjustments, stimulating body rubs, skin brushings, massage, heat/cold immersions, and being wrapped in his Orgone blanket for hours at a time. This was part of his cancer cure treatment, which led to his own incarceration. He had case histories of over 200 cured cancer patients. Dr. Liss is only one of the unsung heroes in the nature healing arts.

Appendix 3

Rest Assured: Parasympathetic Resonance Album

My album *Rest Assured: Parasympathetic Resonance* invites intention to rest, to entrain, to restore, and to re-member how to live within the parasympathetic nervous system. The parasympathetic nervous system is the place that our being can rest, relax, meditate, digest, and assimilate our nutritional needs.

The recording was created with the intention to help the nervous system rest, to encourage rest when the body cannot find rest and seeks it. It is designed for your relaxation listening. Receive and allow the sounds to touch and massage your inner landscape; the power of sound with intention.

The recording is beneficial for relaxation and receiving massage. It supports yoga movement and contemplative meditative listening.

I created this recording by playing, sounding, and listening from my own parasympathetic nervous system to authentically communicate this mending resonance.

For more information and to order visit www.sacredsoundworks.com.

Exercise Overview

Chapter 1

Perception

Chapter 2

Signature Hum

Soothing Hum

The Hum as Resonance
Protection

Chapter 3

Vowel Shaping

Chapter 4

Softening the Jaw with the
Silent AH

The AH Massage

Moving Deeper into AH

Emptying

Reclaiming Our Exhale

The Evolutionary Possibility
of the Exhale

Chapter 5

How to Listen to a Layer

Chapter 6

Aligning and Tuning the Body

Listening to the Rhythms

Chapter 7

Ground Force Reaction—
Plugging In

Ground Force Reaction and the
Heart Field

The Parasympathetic Breath
and Sound

Let Your Gut Brain Talk to Your
Head Brain

Chapter 9

Singing a Love Song to Ourselves

Ask Your Inner Character

Character Formula Laboratory

References

Books

Aston, Judith. *Moving Beyond Posture*. Incline Village, NV: Aston Kinetics, 2007.

Bailey, Alice. *The Unfinished Autobiography*. New York: Lucis Trust, 1951.

Barks, Coleman. *The Essential Rumi*. New York: HarperCollins, 1994.

Beech, Marilyn. *Unexpected Results: Exploring the Edges of Consciousness*. CreateSpace Independent Publishing Platform, 2015.

Buhner, Stephen. *Secret Teachings of Plants*. Rochester, VT: Inner Traditions, 2004.

Conrad, Emilie. *Life on Land*. Berkeley, CA: North Atlantic Books, 2007.

Cordova-Rios, Manuel & Bruce F. Lamb. *Wizard of the Upper Amazon*. Toronto, Canada: McClelland and Stewart Ltd, 1971.

Dodd, Vickie. *Tuning the Blues to Gold: Soundprints*. Boulder, CO: Woven Word Press, 1999.

Eckhart, Meister. *Selected Writings*. New York: Penguin Books, 1995.

Gendlin, Eugene. *Focusing*. New York: Bantam, 1982.

Gershon, Michael M.D. *The Second Brain*. New York: Harper Perennial, 1999.

Gladstar, Rosemary. *The Science & Art of Herbalism* Classic Print Course. Waitsfield, VT: The Science & Art of Herbalism Home Study and Online Course, 2010.

Heline, Corinne. *Music: The Keynote to Human Evolution*. Internet Archive: New Age Press, 1965, 2002.

Henderson, Julie. *Embodying Well-Being*. Self-published. 1999.

Hunt, Dr. Valerie. *Infinite Mind*. Malibu, CA: Malibu Publishing Co, 1989.

Krishnamurti, Jiddu. *Freedom From the Known*. Ojai, CA: Krishnamurti Foundation, 1969.

Narby, Jeremy. *The Cosmic Serpent*. New York: Penguin Putnam Inc., 1998.

Nin, Anais. *Delta of Venus*. Boston, MA: Mariner Books, 2004.

Novalis. *Hymns to the Night*. Brooklyn, NY: Angelico Press, 2020.

Pert, Candace. *Molecules of Emotion*. New York: Simon and Schuster, 1997.

Radocy, Rudolph and David Boyle. *Psychological Foundations of Musical Behavior*. Springfield, IL: Charles C. Thomas Pub Ltd, 2012.

Rolf, Dr. Ida. *Rolfing*. Rochester, VT: Healing Arts Press, 1989.

Solomont, Elide. *You Are Who You Hate*. Burlington, VT: Vantage Press, 1995.

Tiller, William. *Science and Human Transformation*. Walnut Creek, CA: Pavior Publishing, 1997.

Van Dyke, Deborah. *Travelling the Sacred Sound Current: Keys for Conscious Evolution*. Bowen Island, BC, Canada: Sound Current Music, 2001.

CD and Online Resources

Dodd, Vickie. *YouTube Channel*. https://www.youtube.com/sacredsoundworks

———. *Rest Assured: Parasympathetic Resonance*. CD. https://sacredsoundworks.com

———. *Resonance Meditations: A Restorative Journey*. CD. https://sacredsoundworks.com

———. *The Well Cell: Waking up the Amnesia of Wellness*. CD. https://sacredsoundworks.com

Gladstar, Rosemary. *The Science and Art of Herbalism: An Outstanding Herbal Home Study Course*. https://scienceandartofherbalism.com

Laughter Meditation. "Laraaji: Celestial Music Performances and Seriously Playful Laughter Workshops." http://laraaji.blogspot.com

Acknowledgments

I want to acknowledge with deep appreciation the many clients, students, and friends who, 50 years ago, trusted me enough to receive this new work called "Sounding." They had the willingness to be a laboratory for insights gleaned from voice and sound for healing body, mind, and soul. During those first decades, I was granted the opportunity to study, observe, and witness that, yes, sound awakens conscious possibilities.

I am grateful to Christina Castigliano for deciphering and transcribing stacks of hand-written pages. Donna Wolf began the editing process of the manuscript, bringing increased clarity.

Teresa Posakony helped bring the writing into the polished piece of art it is today. She understood the message I wanted to convey with the book. I have much gratitude for her dedication to accuracy and her ability to sense the rhythm, flow, and timing of the words.

I give heartfelt thanks to friends who helped me persevere, read various generations of the manuscript, offered helpful feedback, and kept reminding me that "it works." They include Eric Neurath; Mary Jo Hoven; Sissi Bruch; Kimberly Maroney; Linda Krier; John Galm; Rosemary Gladstar; and Arji Cakouros, who introduced me to my wonderful agent, Joe Kulin, and Sabine Weeke, editorial director of Findhorn Press, publisher of this book.

There are many others through the years, who have now passed on, who encouraged me to trust what I knew about sound and the body, including Kay Gardner, Dr. Mishra, Kali Mai, and William David. I am grateful for my roots and all the mycelium with which I have connected throughout this planet. I know I have left out many loving voices and hands. Please forgive me, and know you are here in my heart with gratitude.

I give all credit to Source and to all frequencies that move throughout this planet in their own rhythms and intentions and aliveness. I am grateful for all the pioneers of sound, mind–body therapies, and spiritual visionaries, who have always been present for each generation that wakes up to these teachings.

About the Author

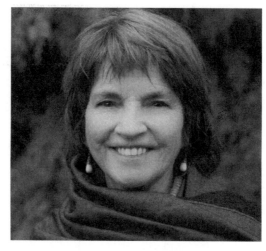

Photo by Eric Neurath

Vickie Dodd, founder of Sacred SoundWorks, is an internationally known pioneer in the field of sound as bodywork. An Aston-Patterning teacher, author, poet, nutritionist, herbalist, workshop leader, and musician, Vickie started using sound as a healing modality in her work with her clients more than 50 years ago.

She has designed a system that integrates emotional memories within the physical body and facilitates the release of long-held emotional distress. Vickie has become one of the most recognized healers and teachers of sound healing worldwide and created sound school trainings in Switzerland, Argentina, and in the USA. She collaborated with Don Campbell in the Institute of Music and Health Education in Boulder, Colorado, and is currently an adjunct faculty member at the Globe Institute in San Francisco. She is the author of *Tuning The Blues To Gold: Soundprints* and has several audio recordings available.

For more information visit: **www.sacredsoundworks.com**